THE FALL OF AN ICON:
PSYCHOANALYSIS AND ACADEMIC PSYCHIATRY

Over the last few decades, academic psychiatry has undergone a revolution. After the Second World War, most department chairs were psychoanalysts who belonged to separate institutes, not subject to the checks and balances of academia, and who did not subscribe to the tenets of scientific medicine. The revolution against psychoanalytic dominance began when a group of psychiatrists developed an evidence-based model that brought psychiatry back into the medical mainstream.

In *The Fall of an Icon*, Joel Paris traces the history of this transition, placing it in the context of current trends in science and medicine. He illustrates the story using interviews with prominent academic psychiatrists in Canada and the United States, and describes his own experiences as a psychiatrist: how he was caught up in the excitement of the psychoanalytic model, how he became disillusioned with it, and how he came to a new and more scientific view of his discipline. This is an essential work for understanding the recent history of psychiatry.

JOEL PARIS is a professor in the Department of Psychiatry at McGill University.

The Fall of an Icon

Psychoanalysis and Academic Psychiatry

JOEL PARIS

UNIVERSITY OF TORONTO PRESS
Toronto Buffalo London

© University of Toronto Press Incorporated 2005
Toronto Buffalo London
Printed in Canada

ISBN 0-8020-3933-2 (cloth)
ISBN 0-8020-3772-0 (paper)

Printed on acid-free paper

Library and Archives Canada Cataloguing in Publication

Paris, Joel, 1940–
Fall of an icon : psychoanalysis and academic psychiatry / Joel Paris.

Includes bibliographical references and index.
ISBN 0-8020-3933-2 (bound). ISBN 0-8020–3772-0 (pbk.)

1. Psychoanalysis – Canada – History. –   2. Psychoanalysis – United
States – History.   3. Psychiatry – Canada – History – 20th century.
4. Psychiatry – United States – History – 20th century.   I. Title.

RC506.P37 2005   616.89′17′0971   C2004-905762-6

University of Toronto Press acknowledges the financial assistance to its
publishing program of the Canada Council for the Arts and the
Ontario Arts Council.

University of Toronto Press acknowledges the financial support for its
publishing activities of the Government of Canada through the
Book Publishing Industry Development Program (BPIDP).

This book is dedicated to Ned Shorter

Contents

Acknowledgments

This book is dedicated to Edward Shorter, professor of the history of Medicine at the University of Toronto. I owe Ned a great deal. The author of a standard text, *A History of Psychiatry* (New York: Wiley, 1998), Ned suggested I should focus this book on academic psychiatry, the setting I know best. He read every chapter several times, each time making valuable suggestions for improvement.

I also received early encouragement for this project from Allan Young, professor in the Faculty of Medicine at McGill University. Roz Paris read the manuscript carefully and gave me very helpful input. Judy Grossman aided me in finding obscure references.

I am grateful to the academic psychiatrists who agreed to be interviewed for this book. Each of them donated valuable time, both in talking to me and in reviewing and correcting my notes from the interviews. Their names are listed at the end of this volume.

The reader may note that all the psychiatrists I formally interviewed work in the United States. Most of the changes in psychiatry I describe in this book began there, and then spread to Canada. I needed more direct knowledge of how events unfolded south of the border. At the same time, I have related many personal experiences and developments that belong to the history of Canadian psychiatry. I would therefore like to acknowledge my teachers at McGill University, as well as colleagues in Montreal and elsewhere in Canada who have enriched my understanding of psychiatry over several decades.

THE FALL OF AN ICON:
PSYCHOANALYSIS AND ACADEMIC PSYCHIATRY

Introduction

One could fill a library with all the books ever written about Freud and psychoanalysis. The analytic movement was one of the keystones of twentieth-century thought. Yet, as many writers have noted,[1] the influence of psychoanalysis has been waning over recent decades. To explain this decline, some have focused on the problems of analysis as a theory of mind.[2] Others have emphasized its limitations as a therapy.[3]

This book will tell another story, one that is not widely known. After the Second World War, psychoanalysis dominated academic psychiatry. Forty years ago, the most influential departmental chairs in North America were trained psychoanalysts.[4] Many prominent teachers in psychiatry belonged to an even more exclusive inner elite: training analysts who supervised candidates at independent 'institutes.' For a time, psychiatry as a discipline became almost indistinguishable from psychoanalysis. Graduates of the top residency programs aspired to become either psychotherapists or fully trained analysts.

Beginning in the 1970s, psychoanalysis began to fall out of favour. Today, at major North American universities, chairs of departments and senior professors are likely to be researchers in the neurosciences.[5] Graduates of residency programs prepare for careers in which psycho-pharmacology is a primary skill.

This book will document this change, explaining how and why it happened. I will tell the story using both data and narrative material. I have collected reminiscences from academic psychiatrists around North America, and will also illustrate my ideas with personal experiences – describing how I, in common with so many other psychiatrists of my generation, fell in and out of love with psychoanalysis.

How Psychoanalysis Conquered North America

Psychoanalysis originated in central Europe, but established a new home in America.[6] Ironically, psychoanalysis had less success in Europe, where it was rejected by most academic psychiatrists. Yet the analytic movement obtained great influence on psychiatry in North America.

Americans have always been receptive to new ideas and willing to import them from abroad. As early as 1909, Freud and Jung were invited to lecture at Clark University in Massachusetts. Freud's ideas aroused interest among psychiatrists, but had an even greater impact on the wider culture. Psychoanalysis, with its emphasis on the unconscious and sexuality, had a great appeal for intellectuals of the 1920s.[7] In the artistic community, many creative people either entered analysis or freely made use of its ideas. Analysis in the United States became associated with the culture of Greenwich Village,[8] and its ideas were taken up by political radicals whose lifestyle eschewed sexual repression. W.H. Auden, in an elegy on Freud's death, put it neatly: 'for us, he has now become, not a person, but a climate of opinion.'[9]

Psychoanalysis was more than a theory. It was also a method of therapy that claimed unusual success in a vast array of mental illnesses. This was another reason for its popularity in North America. Many saw this newfangled 'talking cure' as a sign of progress, in contrast to the pessimistic views of European psychiatry. Americans, rejecting Old World values in favour of New World optimism, often prefer to take a 'can do' approach to problems, believing that more things are possible than impossible. Nonetheless, psychoanalysis was not popular everywhere; it had more influence in large cosmopolitan cities,[10] and less impact in the American heartland.

Developments in Canada tend to follow those south of the border. Yet Canadian culture straddles the intellectual divide between European and American traditions. This may explain why the analytic movement influenced psychiatry in Canada somewhat later than it did in the United States.[11] Psychoanalysis established a strong base in Montreal, and then in Toronto – cosmopolitan cities that attracted immigrants and welcomed new ideas. Yet the movement never really gained more than a foothold in the Maritimes or in western Canada. Many of the leaders of Canadian psychiatry in the twentieth century had been trained in England, and brought home the British tradition of hard-headed empiricism.

When Psychoanalysis Dominated Academic Psychiatry

When most leaders of North American psychiatry were psychoanalysts, membership in a analytic society was a ticket to a successful academic career. Students tend to emulate their professors. Many of the best and brightest young psychiatrists, even those who did not primarily intend to practise therapy, entered institutes for training.[12]

This was still the case when I trained in psychiatry in the late 1960s. The chair of the McGill department, Bob Cleghorn, was an analyst (albeit best known for his research in endocrinology). Many of the top teachers were firmly committed to analysis. Quite a few of my fellow residents aspired to the prestige and skill that would come from training at an institute.

For young psychiatrists, a commitment to analytic training required large expenditures of time (another five years past residency) and of money (to pay for a lengthy personal analysis). Then, to rise to the elite status of training analyst, one would have to accrue many additional years of experience, and publish papers about psychoanalysis. It is hardly surprising that those who were willing to jump through all these hoops became ferocious defenders of the cause.

For a whole generation of North American psychiatrists, even for those who never entered the inner circle of the movement, the theory and practice of psychoanalysis shaped their education and their practice. For this reason, graduates from the most prestigious universities did not gravitate towards hospitals and clinics where the sickest patients were seen. Some psychiatrists obtained staff positions in university hospitals, retaining an outside office for private patients. Others spent their entire professional lives conducting office psychotherapy with a highly educated, less seriously ill clientele.[13]

In the United States, psychiatric education has always been controlled by hospitals, and is only nominally under the control of universities. State hospitals tend to draw psychiatrists from less-prestigious training sites. Psychiatrists who did their residency in the public system prepared for a career in which they would either remain within these institutions or work in community clinics serving disadvantaged and chronically ill patients. These practitioners often treated patients who were either unsuitable for therapy or who could not afford it. Even in Canada, where psychiatric training is firmly under the control of universities, the results were much the same. In both countries, state or provincial hospitals provided an entry point into the system for foreign graduates who had less influence or impact on the academic world.

Psychoanalysts, who were often the leaders of psychiatry, limited their own practices to high-functioning patients. This was an ethical paradox that contradicted medical tradition. In most specialities, senior physicians, particularly professors, take on the treatment of severely ill patients, as well as patients who have failed to recover under the care of less-expert clinicians. But in psychiatry, the sickest cases were often left to a second level of practitioners outside of the academic community. In an influential critique, the American psychiatrist Fuller Torrey described this situation as 'the abandonment of the mentally ill.'[14]

Standard textbooks define the boundaries of academic disciplines. As a medical student at McGill University in 1962, I was asked to buy a textbook of psychiatry written by two Philadelphia analysts, Spurgeon English and Stuart Finch.[15] This book focused almost exclusively on psychoanalytic theory and practice, giving only a brief nod to recent developments in pharmacology, such as antipsychotics and antidepressants.

Medical practice depends on a base of scientific knowledge. Forty years ago, North American psychiatry had a weak biological tradition, and practitioners had limited knowledge about the brain. As an undergraduate psychology student in 1959, I wrote a term paper on the biology of schizophrenia. After spending many hours in the library, I handed in a comprehensive review with one hundred references. To repeat this task today, I would have to read journal articles numbered in the tens of thousands.[16]

The state of knowledge at the time made it possible for psychoanalysts within psychiatry to espouse a purely psychological theory of schizophrenia.[17] In the postwar era, biological theories were associated with therapeutic pessimism, while psychoanalysis was vastly optimistic. The problem was that excluding or dismissing biological factors in disease isolated psychiatry from medicine, creating an intellectual gulf with other specialists, who reacted by viewing the entire field with suspicion. Most medical specialists were also sceptical about the therapeutic claims of psychoanalysis. Psychiatry did not gain much clout within medicine until research actually led to effective treatments for mental illness.

Until about thirty years ago, the majority of psychoanalysts were psychiatrists.[18] Although Freud had favoured 'lay analysis,'[19] the American Psychoanalytic Association wanted to raise its prestige through links with medicine and, accordingly, exclude most non-medical applicants.[20] As a result, separate institutes for psychologists, as well as a rival organization, the American Academy of Psychoanalysis, emerged. The American Psychoanalytic Association's policy eventually changed – after a successful lawsuit from psychologists, but also when applications from psychiatrists to its institutes began to dry up.

Today, psychologists and social workers are gradually replacing psychiatrists within the ranks of psychoanalysis. One might think that this development could lead to the grounding of analytic ideas in a new intellectual base. However, psychoanalysis never attained the same level of influence on university departments of psychology as on psychiatry. Academic psychology had a very different scientific tradition. While some departments sponsored clinical training programs influenced by an analytic paradigm, most leaned towards behaviourism, and behaviour therapy became clinical psychology's unique niche. Based on learning theory, behaviour therapy had been developed by prominent academic psychologists such as Britain's Hans Eysenck.[21] Clinical psychology aimed to base its training on scientific principles, and most practising psychologists were expected to earn a PhD,[22] gaining at least some exposure to research.

In psychiatry, psychoanalysis was most dominant in the larger universities, as reflected in the number of academic chairs with analytic training and the disproportionate prominence of psychoanalysts as teachers.[23] This skew was also apparent outside academia: by the 1960s, as many as a third of practising psychiatrists had analytic training.[24] As late as 1988, over 20 per cent of American psychiatrists were members either of the orthodox American Psychoanalytic Association or of its heterodox sibling, the American Academy of Psychoanalysis.[25]

Psychoanalysis and Medical Science

In the past, studying medicine was like going to a trade school. We learned how to be physicians by apprenticing ourselves to masters whom we imitated. In contrast, contemporary medicine prides itself on being *evidence-based.* New treatments are based on the latest developments in science, and are expected to undergo careful empirical testing.[26]

While most people take it for granted that medical treatments should be rooted in scientific findings, this is actually a recent development. A professor in the humanities, when I informed him of the existence of a major movement favouring evidence-based medicine, asked me how medicine could ever have *not* been based on evidence. I had to explain that clinical practice has often been more of an art than a science.

Medical training has traditionally been divided into basic sciences (based on formal scientific methods) and clinical sciences (based on the experience of physicians). By the second or third year of training, students move from the hard-science atmosphere of the laboratory to the rough-and-ready world of the clinic.

When I was a medical student in the 1960s, the divide between science and practice was broad. I heard very little about clinical trials. Instead, guidelines for treatment were based on the experience of the most experienced practitioners, that is, our teachers. When a professor stated something to be true, students bowed to his superior expertise. In this atmosphere, treatments based on conjecture and clinical acumen were not especially aberrant. Medicine has always relied on observation to understand disease, and in this tradition physicians tended to draw broad conclusions from single cases. Freud, an acute observer and a great generalizer, did not differ dramatically from his medical contemporaries.

Today, single-case observations have been relegated to the letters column of medical journals. No one can publish without hard data to back up their ideas. Science plays a central role in the understanding of disease, and evidence-based medicine is the guiding principle for practice. Medicine relies on experimentally proven theories, systematic measurements in large cohorts of patients, and empirical assessments of therapeutic interventions. All these principles are strongly supported by universities and by prominent medical journals. Students can be (and are encouraged to be) sceptical and can challenge their professors – as long as they can find evidence in the literature for a contrary point of view. New evidence can more readily overthrow old theories. Nothing is taken for granted, and all treatments must prove their efficacy.

Internal medicine and surgery were the first specialties to integrate these principles. Naturally, psychiatry did not want to be left behind. Many of its leaders were no longer satisfied to have colleagues view them as a fringe movement within medicine, humanistic in spirit but hopeless as a scientific enterprise. At the same time, the development of psychopharmacology moved psychiatry back into the mainstream.[27]

Thus, psychoanalysis, which developed in a time when medicine was semi-scientific, belongs to an earlier era of medical practice, relying largely on clinical acumen and accumulated experience. In medicine, that approach has become an anachronism. Yet psychoanalysts have shown great resistance to these changes.

In medicine, no one would think of quoting the views of experts such as Sir William Osler (1849–1919), the world-famous Canadian physician who dominated medicine a hundred years ago.[28] Yet more than sixty years after the death of Freud, analysts have been unable to shake off his influence. Until recently, it was *de rigueur* for most articles in analytic journals to reference Freud's papers, collected into a heavy set of volumes called the *Standard Edition*.[29] This level of conservatism, along with a resistance to building bridges to science, led psychoanalysis into intellectual stagnation.

Today, young psychiatrists are more likely to be excited by new and exciting developments at the cutting edge of science. The Human Genome Project is only the most dramatic example. An explosion of knowledge in the neurosciences has had enormous influence on clinical psychiatry. Research has defined the function of many brain areas and identified an increasingly large number of neurotransmitters. Imaging techniques and brain scans produce dramatic pictures that actually seem to 'visualize' thought.[30]

As the prestige and the romance formerly attached to psychoanalysis have been transferred to the neurosciences, the way to advancement in academia now lies through scientific research. To obtain a position in university psychiatry departments, an analytic training is considered to be, if anything, a drawback. For this reason, ambitious young psychiatrists have little interest in becoming psychoanalysts. Instead, they look for research training to advance their careers. As Chair of Psychiatry at McGill, I have hired thirty young psychiatrists, among whom only two were taking analytic training. The picture is not much different at other universities.

Today, psychiatrists want to be as scientifically grounded as internists or surgeons. Contemporary medicine is positivistic, accepting only what is measurable. Psychoanalysts had believed that empathy and introspection could provide privileged access to the mind. Today, such access may be more likely to be found in PET scans of the human brain.

For psychoanalysis to survive in this climate, its theories and therapy need to be 'operationalized,' that is, presented in a fashion that allows for empirical testing. Systematic reviews of the research literature have shown that the scientific evidence for Freud's theoretical formulations is thin. Nor has analytic treatment been demonstrated to be consistently or uniquely effective. This book will show that, in spite of the enormous time and resources required to complete an analysis, empirical research on the analytic method has been scarce, and that those studies that have been published have yielded disappointing results.

Ironically, psychoanalysts had claimed to have developed a *scientific* method that provides access to the unconscious mind. Freud, and those who followed him, appropriated the prestige of science to support their theories. Yet psychoanalysis fails to meet the normal criteria for an empirically based discipline. As Karl Popper, a prominent philosopher of science, pointed out,[31] the basic elements of the scientific method require the testing and discarding of conjectures and hypotheses. These procedures have been absent from psychoanalysis, where little is tested and past ideas are rarely discarded.

The analytic movement has reacted in various ways to these criticisms. Some practitioners have rejected science, while others have attempted to rewrite its ground rules. Thus, it has been claimed that the analytic method, which uses clinical material to generate hypotheses, is scientific in its own right.[32] This point of view has been effectively rebutted by the philosopher Adolf Grunbaum,[33] who pointed out how clinical evidence is shaped by the context of treatment. For psychoanalysis to be scientific, it must apply scientific methods. As we will see, only in recent years have a few practitioners, somewhat belatedly, begun to conduct serious research on the theory and methods of psychoanalysis.

Psychoanalysis in the Marketplace

Like any other service, psychoanalysis exists in a marketplace. It has to compete with treatments that claim to offer the same results in less time, and with less expenditure. Competition means that patients are less readily convinced that they should undertake a treatment that may require years of their time and use up a large proportion of their income.

As we will see, psychoanalysis has had to compete with drugs, for market share. Psychopharmacological agents have been shown to do many things that analysis cannot. Moreover, a large number of competing psychotherapies have been developed over the years. While most were based on nothing but the claims of their practitioners, this situation has begun to change.

The most influential psychological treatment today is not psychoanalysis, but cognitive-behavioural therapy (CBT),[34] developed by a former analyst (Aaron Beck of Philadelphia). There are several reasons why CBT was able to move into the niche once occupied by psychoanalysis. First, it developed its own theory and technology. Second, CBT is brief and practical. Third, CBT built research on effectiveness into its model from the very beginning. Fourth, CBT has demonstrated its usefulness in almost every condition that psychiatrists treat. While CBT may also run the danger of being oversold, it addresses the needs of practitioners in a way that analysis did not.

Insurance coverage is another key factor affecting the viability of psychoanalysis. In Washington, DC, full analysis had once been covered by government plans, which encouraged a large number of government employees to undergo treatment.[35] Today, both public and private plans resist funding extended and expensive treatments. Insurance companies, unimpressed with results and concerned about costs, have cut back drastically on most psychotherapy benefits.

In the United States, Health Maintenance Organizations have severely undermined the practice of psychotherapy.[36] HMOs are unwilling to pay for more than a few sessions, a policy that actively discourages the practice of almost any form of talking therapy. This policy is irrational, given the strong evidence for the effectiveness of these interventions, at least in the short term.[37] My American colleagues tell me they cannot practise psychotherapy under such conditions, and are forced to seek out patients who can pay. And the purchasers of such psychotherapy services are not particularly interested in lying on a couch several times a week. Even in the relatively friendly environment of New York City, analysts can no longer find enough patients to fill an office practice.[38]

In Canada, provincial health plans have put few restrictions on the length of psychotherapy. (In Ontario, even formal psychoanalysis by psychiatrists has been funded, although most analysts charge supplementary fees that put the treatment out of reach for many consumers.) Yet even under this liberal policy, few patients seek out extended forms of treatment. In any case, only psychiatrists are paid for by government insurance, and few carry large therapy practices.[39] Thus, the ultimate effect is similar to that in the United States: analytic treatment is generally unavailable for Canadians unless one has the money to pay for it.

In the United States, private hospitals used to offer psychoanalytic treatment on their wards. Today, these programs have had either to close or to radically redefine their missions. The most recent and dramatic example occurred when the prestigious Menninger Clinic in Topeka, Kansas, facing financial ruin, had to close down and move its operations to Baylor University in Houston, Texas.[40] In Canada, a few hospital-based programs admitted patients for analytic therapy, but most of these have closed. Owing to severe restrictions on in-patient admissions imposed by provincial governments, long-term admissions designed for intensive psychotherapy have disappeared.

Yet a shift in market forces is not the only reason for the decline of psychoanalysis. Well before the HMO era, a comparison of two surveys of practice in New Haven (in 1950 and 1978),[41] found that fewer patients over time were being referred either for psychoanalysis or for analytic psychotherapy. Thus, economics cannot be the whole story as to why fewer people today seek to be analyzed. When patients are convinced they need an expensive treatment, such as cardiac surgery, they will spend money to obtain it. In the past, people who 'believed' in analysis were willing to pay for it out of pocket, often at great sacrifice.

After all, psychoanalysis reached the height of its dominance in the 1950s and 1960s, an era in which most patients had little if any insurance. The going rate at the time, about $25 an hour, was steep. Yet I knew many who believed so strongly in the unique efficacy of analysis that they were willing to take on an extra job, or even go into debt, to finance treatment. For those who believed in it, only analysis could radically change one's life, and as it was well worth the sacrifice. For analysts, patients not willing to make these commitments might be considered 'resistant.' To be analysed was a badge of honour, while a failure to undergo treatment was a sign of moral weakness.

Today, psychoanalytic ideas no longer command the same level of belief. Opposition to Freud's theories has become common knowledge, repeatedly discussed in newspapers and magazines, and on television. At the same time, the media trumpets every advance in biological psychiatry, from genetic associations to PET scans. As analytic theories lose their cultural dominance, the average person today is more likely to attribute psychological distress to a 'chemical imbalance' than to a repressed trauma.

As I will show in this book, the most serious problem for analysis has been that its failure to keep its promises. Disillusionment with therapeutic results has definitely contributed to a change in the public image of psychoanalysis. Once seen as a uniquely powerful method of treating the mentally ill, analysis has not been proved effective for severely disturbed patients.

Some psychoanalysts have denied this failure. They have been trained to cope with any lack of results by making treatments longer and longer, in the hope of achieving more. Analysts have always believed that patients need to be 'fully analyzed' before being discharged. It is therefore not surprising that, today, the average length of an analysis, which in its early days could be completed in a few months, is six years.[42] As documented in a study conducted at the Menninger Clinic,[43] some patients remain in treatment for their entire lives. Freud was the first to note that analysis is, by its very nature, interminable.[44] The image of endless treatment may be a standard joke for Woody Allen, but it is also a powerful negative advertisement for entering analysis in the first place.

The reality of the marketplace has led psychoanalysis to stop seeing itself as a first-line therapy. On the web site of the American Psychoanalytic Association,[45] prospective patients are advised to consider analysis only if they have chronic problems that have failed to respond to briefer treatment. Even so, entering on a six-year analysis, with sessions several times a week, and at a cost of tens of thousands of dollars, is not for everyone.

Patients might be expected to make massive investments in medical treatments that have strong supporting evidence for their efficacy. For psychoanalysis, such data does not exist. Psychotherapy is generally effective in the short term, and patients who do not respond to brief interventions can benefit from continuing treatment for up to a year.[46] But research has never shown that therapies lasting *many* years accomplish more.

How the Story Will Be Told

Very few books have been published describing the place of psychoanalysis in academic psychiatry. The best such volume, Nathan Hale's *The Rise and Crisis of Psychoanalysis in the United States*[47] brings the story up to 1985. But a great deal has happened since then.

I cannot claim that this book covers every aspect of a changing picture. However, my role as an academic department chair provides me with an opportunity to obtain an 'inside story' of how psychoanalysis lost its hold on psychiatry. Still, I did not want to limit the story to my own experience or to my own university. I therefore conducted formal interviews with professors of psychiatry at several large American medical schools. These interviews, supplemented by less-formal contacts with colleagues, in both Canada and the United States, provided narrative data that helped me reach general conclusions about the state of academic psychiatry in North America.

The first part of the book, 'Hegemony,' describes how psychoanalysis attained and, for many years maintained, its dominance in academic psychiatry. Using examples from various universities, I show how the analytic movement gained and then lost its influence.

The second part, 'Challenge,' examines how psychoanalysis was brought into question, and how its challengers succeeded in ending its hegemony. The counter-revolution against analysis, which began in a Missouri medical school, led to the development of the third edition of the *Diagnostic and Statistical Manual of Mental Disorders*, DSM-III,[48] a new defining paradigm for North American psychiatry. Other challenges to psychoanalysis came from the psychopharmacological revolution and from the development of alternative methods of psychotherapy.

The third part of the book, 'Decline,' concerns the future of psychoanalysis. This section surveys the contemporary scene in academic psychiatry, in which evidence-based medicine is now the predominant paradigm. In the 'Afterword,' I explore how cultural change might account for the popularity of psychoanalysis in its heyday, and also help to explain its decline.

Part One

HEGEMONY

chapter 1

Psychoanalysis and Psychiatry

Psychiatry and Medicine

Contemporary psychiatry has a respected and secure place within medicine. But this has not always been the case. During the heyday of psychoanalysis, medical specialists reacted with suspicion to psychiatrists, who were not often seen as 'real doctors.' In the 1960s, many physicians expressed contempt for psychiatry, largely because they saw it as more or less synonymous with psychoanalysis.

Paradoxically, medical students chose psychiatry for this very reason. Becoming a psychiatrist was seen as the only way to become a physician who cared about the mind and the soul. Medical schools of the 1960s had little place for humanistic ideals. Most of the curriculum was dryly technical. Family medicine had not yet emerged as a separate field. Students who wanted to understand people almost *had* to go into psychiatry. In those halcyon days, the field was young, exciting, and different. In my own class, McGill '64, recruitment into psychiatry stood at 15 per cent. This high level was duplicated in many schools across North America at the time. Today the numbers never go higher than 5 per cent, hovering around 2–3 per cent.[1]

Many psychiatrists, particularly those who became analytically oriented, had already established career goals before entering medical school. Others chose psychiatry during medical school, often after positive experiences with inspiring teachers. Still others turned to psychiatry after working unhappily in another specialty. But any medical student who made the decision to become a psychiatrist had to endure criticism from teachers and peers. Internists and surgeons saw psychiatry as a fringe area with little scientific merit. Teachers accused students interested in the field of abandoning medicine, referring sarcastically to its practitioners as 'witch doctors.'

Even today, if one were to judge what contemporary psychiatry is from *New Yorker* cartoons, the typical practitioner still seems to be a bearded man writing copious notes behind a patient on a couch. The perception that psychiatry and psychoanalysis are identical is an anachronism, but was far from invalid in the 1960s. In my own graduating class, half of those who chose psychiatry took formal training in psychoanalysis, while most of the others practised analytically oriented therapy.

The Two Psychiatries

Fifty years ago, two professors at Yale, August Hollingshead, a sociologist, and Fritz Redlich, a psychiatrist, described psychiatry as divided into two cultures.[2] They noted that there were two types of practitioner in New Haven. A 'directive-organic' group who wore white coats, prescribed medication, and tended to be old-stock New Englanders. The other group, which they termed 'analytic-psychological,' wore sport jackets, preferred talking therapy, and tended to come from immigrant families.

Cultural factors were important in choosing sides. Psychoanalysis had been founded by a Jewish doctor, and most of its early adherents were Jewish. As shown in a survey from the mid-1960s,[3] committed psychotherapists, whether trained as psychiatrists, psychologists, or social workers, were demographically similar to but unrepresentative of the general population. At a time when most Americans were Protestants, and only 3 per cent were Jews, about a third of all psychotherapists were of Jewish background, with most having eastern European roots.

When I began residency in 1968, psychiatry was clearly divided in two. Mental-hospital work was traditionally medical and drug-oriented. Even so, by this time, hospitals were becoming more attractive than in the past. Psychopharmacology was developing rapidly, and I was exposed to one of its pioneers: Heinz Lehmann, a German émigré working at McGill University. The advances in drug treatment in that period were truly revolutionary. For the first time in the history of psychiatry, psychiatrists had effective agents to treat schizophrenia and depression. Patients given these drugs often improved rapidly.

Ten years previously, in 1958, as an undergraduate psychology student, I had spent weekends volunteering at a large mental hospital, Ypsilanti State, in Michigan. Most of the patients were warehoused and left largely untreated. A man suffering from paranoid schizophrenia sat in a corner writing endless notes. A woman with catatonic schizophrenia stood paralysed in the corridor, holding the same position for days. Antipsychotic drugs were being used for the first time, but were prescribed in very low dosages. As psychiatrists became more expert in using the new agents, most of these severely ill patients became treatable. Ypsilanti State, which had four thousand beds in the 1950s, gradually shrank; it closed down entirely during the 1990s.

As early as the 1950s, evidence was gathering to support the concept that brain pathology was behind mental illness. Research into hallucinogenic drugs suggested that one could mimic psychosis with certain chemicals, and one investigator even reported that when spiders were given LSD, they spun 'crazy' webs.[4] But psychopharmacology remained an empirical discipline. No one knew how and where these drugs worked in the brain. It was only when these questions began to be answered through neurobiology that the field earned increased scientific respectability.

Analytic-psychological psychiatry was another world. Instead of being based on scientific method, practice was rooted in the clinical tradition. Analysis was believed to provide access to the unconscious mind. While this claim was never backed up by data, the general public was in awe of the technique's purported capacity to understand the psyche. Psychiatrists or psychiatric residents can be asked at parties whether they could read other people's minds. This belief is not entirely irrational, given that there is such a thing as clinical skill and acumen. But psychiatrists have a simple secret: they have the right to ask probing questions, gaining information within ten minutes to which a patient's long-time friends and intimates never obtain access.

Two Psychiatries and Two Teachers

The two psychiatries had different training programs.[5] Forty years ago, before the development of national guidelines for psychiatric training, these differences could be dramatic, particularly in the United States. Residents at state hospitals spent most of their time treating psychotic patients. In general hospitals dominated by psychoanalysis, residents might spend most of their time conducting psychotherapy on less severely ill patients. These polarities reflected the two-tier system of American psychiatry. The sickest and the poorest patients were seen in state hospitals and community clinics. Teaching hospitals associated with universities were not always interested in these cases.

Medical schools teach psychiatry at multiple sites: general hospitals, children's hospitals, state hospitals, private hospitals, and community clinics. Each setting treats a unique population. I was fortunate to train in Canada, where the system, monitored by the Royal College of Physicians and Surgeons, encouraged me to see every kind of patient and to be taught by every type of teacher.[6] In the United States, however, residents training in psychiatry received most of their education in one, or at most two, clinical settings.

I began the first year of my residency in a psychiatric hospital. My most important teacher during that formative year was Heinz Lehmann. An exemplary 'directive-organic' psychiatrist, Lehmann, born in 1911 in Berlin, came to Canada in 1938. (Lehmann was only half-Jewish, but his decision to emigrate undoubtedly saved his life.)

Lehmann first became interested in psychiatry as a precocious adolescent, reading Freud cover to cover. Later, he rejected analytic ideas, largely on theoretical grounds. Heinz Lehmann was an idealist who decided to devote his career to the care of the severely mentally ill. As an immigrant doctor, his best chance for a job was at a mental hospital, and that is where he spent most of his career.

In 1944, a department of psychiatry was created at McGill under the leadership of the American psychiatrist Ewen Cameron. Lehmann disapproved of many of Cameron's ideas, and kept his distance, happy to work several miles away. (In the 1950s Cameron was infamous for conducting 'brain-washing' experiments on patients, the results of which are still under litigation fifty years later.) Lehmann lived on the hospital grounds in a small house, owned no car, and got around by bicycle. He made daily rounds on hundreds of psychotic patients under his care. On Christmas morning Lehmann would tour the entire hospital, giving holiday greetings to every patient.

Heinz Lehmann died at the age of eight-seven in 1999. He had been a late bloomer who only began to publish research in middle age. Replicating earlier work from Europe that demonstrated the efficacy of antipsychotic and antidepressant drugs, he became a true pioneer. Unlike his psychoanalytic colleagues, most of whom remained immersed in an oral culture, Lehmann published hundreds of data-based articles. As one of the founders of psychopharmacology, he will be remembered for years to come.

Lehmann had little to do with psychoanalysts, and his comments about them could be dismissive, such as 'They seem to be more interested in their theories than in curing disease.' In his view, psychoanalysis was an inefficient method that gave more satisfaction to the analyst than to the patient.

In spite of my early exposure to Lehmann, I wanted to learn about psychoanalysis. I spent the next two years of my residency at the Jewish General Hospital, which was known for its strong analytical orientation. The buzz among the resident group was that this was an exciting, cutting-edge place to train. The chief of psychiatry was Henry Kravitz, a man of great charisma and strong rhetorical skills. Born in Poland but brought up in Canada, Kravitz was a typical example of the analytical-psychological psychiatrist. Although he was a training analyst, Kravitz chose to focus his career on hospital work. That decision was made in the 1950s, when psychoanalysts were beginning to dominate the teaching of psychiatry, and when analytic methods were being extended to treat psychotic patients.

'Rounds with Kravitz' closely resembled an analytic session. The hour began with a fair amount of undigested information. The resident making the case presentation had to be sure to include details about the patient's childhood. Kravitz, tapping gently on his pipe, would begin by listening without saying much. Knowing what was to come, few other staff members would venture an opinion before the Chief spoke. Then, about ten minutes before the end of the hour, Kravitz brilliantly drew the strands of the case together into a coherent narrative. Heads around the room would nod, partly in agreement and partly in awe at the quality of the performance.

In 1980, McGill organized a special debate between Heinz Lehmann and Henry Kravitz concerning the future of psychiatry. Lehmann, presenting views that were later published,[7] argued that psychiatry had to 'bite the bullet' and accept the new realities of mental-health care delivery. Psychiatrists, in whom society had invested expensive years of training, should not be spending much of their time conducting psychotherapy, since this technique does not require a medical degree. Instead, they should focus on activities that make use of their unique skills: emergency treatment of severely ill patients, in-patient care for the sickest patients, as well as out-patient management of patients with unstable psychoses and intractable depression. In addition, psychiatrists should reach out to the larger mental-health community, and spend more time providing consultations: to family doctors, to psychologists and social workers, and to therapists of all persuasions.

Kravitz had a very different view of the future. Psychiatrists must continue to make use of their special skills in understanding psychopathology and the workings of the mind. Were they to become psychopharma-cologists and consultants, as Lehmann recommended, they would abandon patients needing the skills of a specialist. Even when drugs were necessary, psychiatrists, trained in both medicine and therapy, would be in a unique position to treat severely ill patients.

At the time this debate was held, I was inclined to support Kravitz's position. Over the years, I gravitated to Lehmann's point of view, and psychiatry as a whole moved in the same direction. As will be discussed later in this book, the new generation of psychiatrists is less interested in psychotherapy, and most now spend a majority of their time treating psychotic and severely depressed patients.

My experience with the two psychiatries was typical of university-based residency training in the late 1960s. Yet the controversy about what a psychiatrist should be is still alive. Analysts are deeply upset about what has happened to psychiatry. Today, few defend training psychiatrists to conduct office practices with purely neurotic patients. Instead, they espouse a broad model of treatment in which psychiatrists play a unique role because of their skills in both drug treatment and psychotherapy. A recent article in the American Journal of Psychiatry by two prominent psychoanalysts (Glen Gabbard and John Gunderson)[8] argued that mental health care is becoming unnecessarily fragmented between physicians and therapists, while psychiatrists provide comprehensive care that is integrated and cost-effective. (This may be true, but psychiatrists are expensive, and there will never be enough of them to meet the demand.)

Psychoanalysis and Psychiatry after the Second World War

By the 1920s, psychoanalysis was well established in America.[9] Then an exodus of psychoanalysts from Europe during the Nazi era greatly strengthened the movement. Its earlier adherents, such as Abraham Brill and Frederick Putnam, were overshadowed by influential émigrés such as Franz Alexander, Otto Fenichel, Heinz Hartmann, and Margaret Mahler. Quickly adapting to the local context, these eminent teachers attracted new recruits, making psychoanalysis into a truly American movement.

The postwar period in America was a unique historical moment, full of hope and promise. Psychiatry enjoyed a dramatically expanding social influence, and psychoanalysis had something to offer to both psychiatries. Clinicians still had a limited ability to treat patients, a problem that applied to both psychiatries. Hospital-based practitioners saw patients suffering from illnesses, such as schizophrenia and manic depression, for which they had no effective treatment. Office-based practitioners saw patients with milder illnesses, and were more inclined to prescribe psychotherapy, yet lacked effective remedies for common complaints such as anxiety and depression. Outside the framework of psychoanalysis, talking therapy lacked a theoretical structure and had no well-described method. In practice, psychotherapies were given on a 'hit and miss' basis. Analytic therapy at least offered a coherent frame-work for conducting office psychotherapy on neurotic patients. In pri-vate mental hospitals, psychoanalysts were also experimenting with the treatment of psychosis. These methods seemed to offer hope for patients long considered incurable.

Caring for hospitalized psychotic patients was an enormous chal-lenge. In the absence of useful alternatives, 'great and desperate cures' emerged.[10] After the war, strong claims were made for the effectiveness of prefrontal lobotomy. This treatment earned a Nobel Prize for Egas Moniz, the Portuguese neurologist who had originally advocated it, as well as honours for Walter Freeman, the American psychiatrist who pop-ularized lobotomy, travelling from hospital to hospital to demonstrate the procedure. But the results of psychosurgery quickly turned sour, and were in any case made obsolete by the greater effectiveness of drugs. While less-radical neurosurgical procedures might still be used for refractory cases, for most clinicians, even the mention of lobotomy elicits a shudder.

The postwar era also saw the expanded use of electro-convulsive therapy (ECT), first introduced by Italian psychiatrists in the 1930s. Although originally developed as a treatment for schizophrenia, its results in that disease were transient. On the other hand, ECT was highly effective in severe depressions.[11] Unlike lobotomy, this procedure is still widely used today. ECT only became controversial because of overuse. In an era without antidepressant drugs, psychiatrists were tempted to treat almost *any* depression with electroconvulsive therapy.

As an idealistic young resident, I did not know what to make of ECT. (This was even before it was satirized in the popular film *One Flew Over the Cuckoo's Nest*.) Then, while training in a large psychiatric hospital, I obtained experience in prescribing and administering the treatment. The very first patient I treated, a middle-aged man with depression, responded rapidly, recovering after only a few treatments. However ECT works, its effects can be dramatic.

In the pre-psychopharmacological era, ECT was almost the only truly effective treatment psychiatrists had. Almost the only drugs that could be used to calm psychotic patients were barbiturates. Without specific treatment, patients often languished for months to years on wards. General hospitals were beginning to open psychiatry units, but these settings were mainly used for patients with less-severe illnesses. Psychotic patients, often indigent, and less interesting to many psychiatrists, were quickly transferred to the mental hospital, which was also left with responsibility for long-term care.

In this context, psychiatric practice could sometimes become experimental, attempting at all costs to counter therapeutic nihilism. Ewen Cameron,[12] the founder of the Department of Psychiatry at McGill, began giving patients long courses of electro-convulsive therapy, which reduced them, at least temporarily, to a state of complete helplessness. Cameron believed that his method, like the regression produced by psychoanalysis, could provide an opportunity to teach patients coping skills by forcing them to start from scratch.

Experimental methods were generally used for sicker patients. There were no effective biological treatments for the most common disorders seen in practice. In the absence of viable alternatives, psychoanalysis won out. Analytic therapy was likely to be prescibed for depression, anxiety, and personality disorders. Even so, there was an economic barrier to treatment. If they could afford it, patients would be seen privately. If not, they would receive a lower standard of care at clinics in the hospital or the community. Moreover, as long as the sickest patients were being sent to mental hospitals, academic psychiatrists, centred in general hospitals, could focus on patients with less-severe pathology.

The conquest of academic psychiatry by psychoanalysis did not come about until after the Second World War. Before that, although some analysts had joined university departments, the leadership of North American psychiatry remained sceptical and uncommitted.

The Swiss-American psychiatrist Adolf Meyer (1857–1950), working at Johns Hopkins University, had enormous influence on psychiatry before the Second World War.[13] Meyer was a mentor to many departmental chairs in both the United States and Canada. His perspective on mental illness was largely psychological, and he even advocated talking therapy for schizophrenia. Thus, though Meyer remained a sceptic about Freud's treatment, he set the stage for its triumph.

As early as the 1920s, the Menninger family had opened a psychiatric hospital in Kansas offering treatment programs based on analytic principles.[14] Karl Menninger, who became one of the deans of American psychiatry, became well known by the general public through his books, and also earned great respect from psychiatrists around the world. (When I attended the 1971 meeting of the World Psychiatric Association in Mexico City, his very entrance to give a talk drew a standing ovation.)

Karl's brother, William, although not formally trained as an analyst, was a strong sympathizer of the movement. William's crucial role in American psychiatry began during the Second World War, when he was put in charge of psychiatric services for the military and made a brigadier general. During the war, analysts such as Roy Grinker of Chicago, who went on to become a leader of American psychiatry, developed methods for the treatment of psychiatric casualties that gave a Freudian spin to the war's effects. In a widely read book, Grinker and Spiegel[15] claimed that combat neuroses could be rapidly treated with 'abreaction' (i.e., reliving traumatic experiences), much in the same way as Freud had treated Viennese hysterics in the 1890s.

After the war ended, William Menninger retained the ear of the American government. The Menninger brothers were now in a position to shape the future of psychiatry. In 1946, they created a 'think tank' called the Group for the Advancement of Psychiatry (GAP).[16] Over the years, this organization produced documents, entitled 'GAP reports,' that appeared regularly and that shaped opinion in academic psychiatry. GAP promulgated a humanistic version of psychoanalysis. Its theoretical position was that mental health and illness are on a continuum, and it consistently argued for prevention, community psychiatry, and social activism.

The Menningers were also influential leaders in psychiatric education. For some time, positions for psychiatric trainees had been poorly funded. But in 1946, following an initiative led by William Menninger, the U.S. Congress created a national program for research and psychiatric training. This organization later evolved into the National Institute of Mental Health (NIMH).[17] In this context of expansion, the Menninger Institute in Topeka was perfectly positioned to take the lead. A well-endowed private hospital, it trained a large number of residents, and most of its graduates emerged with a strong analytic orientation, many becoming professors at major American universities.

As will be described in chapter 6, NIMH, at least in its early days, supported psychoanalysis, which was then the leading theory in psychiatry. Universities with analytically oriented programs received grants from

NIMH to pay for the salaries of residents training in psychiatry. In 1955, when a new department of psychiatry was founded at Yeshiva University in New York, the NIMH actually agreed to provide partial funding for residents to undergo personal analyses.

Over the next few decades, the growth of the field and the influence of analysis dramatically changed the profile of psychiatry.[18] In 1940, 67 per cent of psychiatrists had worked in hospitals; this figure fell to 17 per cent by 1956. Residency programs doubled between 1946 and 1956, and the total number of trainees quintupled, while the number of hours in the psychiatric curriculum for subjects related to psychoanalysis quadrupled. This was also the peak time of choice for psychiatry among medical students, reaching an all time high of 12.5 per cent in 1954.

The extent of psychoanalytic influence varied greatly by region.[19] As we will see, psychoanalysis took a long time to become dominant in Canada. In the United States, the movement was always more successful in large cities and coastal regions. The American east coast, with its stronger European orientation, was a preferred point of entry for immigrant analysts. Cities such as New York and Boston had no lack of patients seeking this form of treatment, and major training centres had been organized there by the 1930s. In the American heartland, Chicago, under the charismatic leadership of Freud's disciple Franz Alexander, became another great centre for analytic training. Psychoanalysis was also influential in Los Angeles, where it earned strong allegiance from the film community. In all these cities, the movement had little trouble gaining power and influence in the academic community.

Elsewhere, success was more spotty. The culture of Middle America, rooted in agriculture and religious beliefs, was less receptive to analytic ideas. Outside the enclave created by the Menningers in Kansas, many medical schools remained hostile, even excluding psychoanalysis from their training programs. As we will see, one midwestern department, Washington University in St Louis, later played a crucial role in driving analysis out of academic psychiatry.

Postwar American Psychiatry as Depicted in the Pages of Its Most Prominent Journal

The *American Journal of Psychiatry* is delivered monthly to the thousands of members of the American Psychiatric Association (APA). First published in 1844 (as the *American Journal of Insanity*), it is the most widely read periodical in psychiatry, both in the United States and in Canada.

The 'green journal' (a reference to the long-standing colour of its cover) evolved over the years into a prestigious and powerful scientific publication. Its pages provide a series of historical snapshots illuminating the state of American psychiatry.

We can begin the story in 1944, the 100th anniversary of the APA.[20] The contents of the *American Journal* in that year reflected the times, and many pages were filled with reports about military psychiatry. However, in 1944, the *Journal* could best be described as a collection of opinion pieces and clinical reports. Scientific medicine was still in its infancy. Most articles contained only a few references. Hardly any of them made serious use of statistics. The small smattering of biological papers were unsystematic, although sometimes illustrated with impressive photographs showing microscopic sections of the brain.

In 1944, most studies of psychiatric patients consisted entirely of 'case series.' These papers contained nothing but simple counts of symptoms from consecutive patients seen in a particular clinical setting. Samples were idiosyncratic and unrepresentative. In the absence of systematic comparisons with control groups, results were difficult to interpret. The *Diagnostic and Statistical Manual of Mental Disorders*, the American Psychiatric Association's first guide to categorization, would not be published until 1952.[21] In an era when even DSM-I did not exist, diagnosis was primitive and unreliable. Moreover, there were no controlled studies of treatment methods. (The first clinical trial in medicine, establishing the value of streptomycin for tuberculosis, was not published until 1946.)[22] The reader was expected to accept, almost on faith, claims for success based on the percentage of patients who improved when given a particular treatment.

At this time, the *American Journal* was not dominated by psychoanalysis. From 1931 to 1965, the editor was Clarence B. Farrar, a Hopkins-trained psychiatrist who ran the Toronto Psychiatric Hospital. Farrar was a practical man, much in the tradition of his teacher Adolf Meyer, and the journal reflected his point of view. Thus, in the mid-1940s, the *American Journal of Psychiatry* was publishing only a few articles on psychoanalysis. Freud had only died in 1939, and his movement remained institutionally separate. Psychoanalysts published in their own journals. Psychiatric departments were medical, and anyone who wanted to study analysis had to enrol in an institute.

To mark the hundredth anniversary of the *Journal*, Alan Gregg, a well-known neurologist who advised the Rockefeller Foundation on the funding of medical research, wrote an article entitled 'A Critique of Psychiatry.'[23] Some of Gregg's comments sound familiar sixty years later: psychiatry was having problems obtaining recruits; the field was too isolated from medicine; although over-burdened, the field was too long-suffering to seek support from the public. Gregg only mentioned psychoanalysis in passing, but was dubious about the movement's scientific credentials: 'I cannot escape the impression that psychoanalysts usually resent or spurn requests for proof or experimental verification of their postulates.' Gregg must have been surprised when, only a few years later, the movement virtually took over American psychiatry.

Psychoanalysis and the Psychoses

Psychoanalysis has a tradition of converting clinical observations into causal theories. In the 1950s, when psychoanalysts interested in schizophrenia observed that some of the families of patients were troubled, they developed theories *blaming* these families (especially mothers) for the illness.[24] If schizophrenia was psychogenic, it might be cured by therapy.

As a resident, I observed some of the errors that resulted from this theory. When families were brought in for interviews, even if the parents were not told point-blank that the illness was their fault, they usually got the point. When problems in communication were observed, they were used to confirm current theories about schizophrenia, such as the idea that these parents put their children in a 'double bind'[25] (i.e., damned if you do, and damned if you don't). When marital discord was observed, it was used to prove that the patient (sometimes referred to as the 'identified patient') was only 'a carrier for family pathology.'

No one seemed to consider the obvious alternative that families are terribly affected by having a psychotic child. This is a stressor that interferes with family communication, and can sometimes break up marriages. Today, given the overwhelming evidence that schizophrenia is a disease of the brain,[26] psychiatrists may find it difficult to understand how seriously previous ideas were held. Yet when I trained, claims that family dysfunction is a cause of schizophrenia were arousing great excitement. These theories led to the idea that psychotherapy, or family therapy, might be a cure for the disease.

This story has been beautifully told in a book by Edward Dolnick, *Madness on the Couch*;[27] I need only summarize it briefly here. Freud developed psychoanalysis as a treatment for neurosis, and thought it contraindicated for psychosis.[28] He took it for granted that schizophrenia had an organic component that would not be addressed by talking therapy. Yet after Freud's death, analysts such as Karl Menninger began to suggest that psychosis and neurosis were not essentially different, constituting points on a continuum of severity.[29]

Freud had believed that neurotic symptoms emerge from childhood conflicts occuring between three and five years of age.[30] But what if psychosis were just a more severe form of neurosis, emerging from conflicts at an earlier point of childhood, possibly in infancy? Psychoanalytic therapy might be more difficult with psychotic patients, but not impossible.

As early as the 1920s, American psychiatrist Harry Stack Sullivan[31] had been treating hospitalized psychotic patients, first at New York's Payne Whitney Clinic. But the analytic therapy of schizophrenia really caught fire in the 1950s. One of its best-known practitioners was Frieda Fromm-Reichmann,[32] an immigrant psychoanalyst working at Chestnut Lodge, a private hospital in Maryland. A tiny but highly maternal woman, she was referred to with affection by her students as 'The Great Breast.'

Fromm-Reichmann believed that schizophrenia could be cured with empathy and understanding. Her most famous patient was Joanne Greenberg, who described her therapy in the best-selling novel *I Never Promised You a Rose Garden*.[33] The story was later turned into a successful film (with Bibi Andersson playing a taller, but still sympathetic Fromm-Reichmann) that made the analysis of psychosis into effective drama.

In Greenberg's novel, an adolescent fantasizes about living on another planet. After being admitted to hospital, she gradually gives up this idea, and the care of her sympathetic therapist helps her to return to reality. When the protagonist complains that reality is not superior to her imaginary world, the fictional version of Fromm-Reichmann tells her, 'I never promised you a rose garden.' (In the 1970s, I treated a strikingly similar case, a French-Canadian adolescent who heard voices from an imaginary world, in another galaxy, telling her to kill herself in order to return to a better place.)

Joanne Greenberg's therapy was a success; she went on to a career as a novelist and raised a family. But was Greenberg ever truly psychotic? In a condition called 'borderline personality disorder,' patients can develop, among other symptoms, intense fantasies that can border on psychosis. Yet unlike schizophrenic patients, these people often recover when their life circumstances change.

Tom McGlashan, a colleague of mine from Yale who spent the early years of his career at Chestnut Lodge, carried out a large-scale study on the long-term outcome of patients treated at that hospital.[34] In the

1950s, American psychiatrists had a very broad concept of schizophrenia, which led to a serious over-diagnosis of the disorder. When McGlashan conducted his research study in 1980, he established more precise diagnoses using current (DSM-III) criteria.

On fifteen-year follow-up, schizophrenic patients, in spite of the efforts of therapists like Fromm-Reichmann, fared just as poorly as those treated in traditional mental hospitals. McGlashan reviewed Greenberg's case in detail, and included her in his sample of eighty-seven that met the criteria for borderline personality disorder.[35] The vast majority of patients in that group had improved greatly by the fifteen-year follow-up.

Thus, most cases of psychosis do poorly with analytic treatment, and the few that were successful may not have been psychotic to begin with. This is what we know now. But in the 1950s, therapists such as Harold Searles[36] at Chestnut Lodge, Elvin Semrad[37] at Harvard, Silvano Arieti[38] in New York, and Otto Will[39] at Yale were invited to speak all across the country, and wrote chapters in standard textbooks. Arieti even edited his own textbook of psychiatry.[40] Owing to a heavy Italian accent, Arieti was unimpressive as a speaker. But his theory, that family pathology caused schizophrenia, was very influential.

This level of respect even applied to less-reputable therapists working on the fringe of psychiatry. In the late 1950s, a New York psychiatrist, John Rosen, advocated a form of treatment called 'direct analysis,' which used rather wild 'deep interpretations' to shock patients out of psychosis.[41] Typically, five minutes into an interview, he might be telling patients that they wanted to sleep with their mothers, or with Rosen himself.

Rosen was a showman who impressed many people. I found him to be taken seriously by psychiatrists at sites as disparate as Ypsilanti State and the Jewish General Hospital in Montreal. Years later, it was shown that all Rosen's cures were spurious, and that the patients he treated had not really recovered. Eventually, Rosen lost his licence for physically beating patients at a private house he used for his version of 'therapy.'[42]

I had one personal experience with the psychotherapy of schizophrenia. As a first-year resident assigned to a mental hospital, I was reading Fromm-Reichmann and Searles, and wanted to have some of the same experiences. With the permission of my supervisor (a psychoanalyst), I started seeing a young schizophrenic patient several times a week in therapy. He was a twenty-five-year-old man with chronic delusions who had recently shot himself under the influence of the voices he was hearing. I managed to obtain dramatic changes within a few weeks. He livened up and talked about his problems, and his parents reported that he had learned to water-ski at their Vermont cottage. But this improvement was short lived. After a couple of months, he was back to square one, and I decided to see him less often.

I should have known better. Heinz Lehmann had already told me how he had tried the same sort of thing in the 1950s. A documentary film made at his hospital had also shown that occupational therapy could lead to dramatic (but temporary) improvement in backward cases. Patients got a lot better, and then a lot worse. Schizophrenia was like that. You had to take a long-range view of the problem.

Not everyone in psychiatry learned these lessons. Gradually, however, disappointment with results escalated. In my series of interviews with leading psychiatrists who trained at that time, a theme that emerged repeatedly concerned 'broken promises,' that is, disillusionment about the efficacy of analytic therapy for psychotic patients.

Max Planck, one of the founders of quantum physics, famously remarked that scientists rarely change their minds about their theories, even when confronted with contradictory evidence.[43] Instead, the older generation dies off and is replaced with young people who espouse different ideas.

The analysts who claimed to be able to treat psychotic patients never really changed their minds. Dolnick poignantly described his interview with Theodore Lidz, the once-influential Yale psychiatrist who had advocated a theory that schizophrenia is the result of family dysfunction.[44] Lidz eventually became an exile within his own profession, and died a few years ago without ever admitting that he might have been wrong.

Today, the younger generation of psychiatrists has little interest in analytic treatments for psychosis. Most of my students have never heard of Lidz, or any of the other leaders who were prominent forty years ago. The only current interest in psychological treatment for psychotic patients has come from cognitive-behavioural therapists, who have developed techniques to help patients cope with their daily lives.

In the 1960s, moreover, the search for an analytic cure for schizophrenia even led some therapists to resist using effective pharmacological therapy. On the basis of their theoretical principles, analysts in the early 1960s thought that one should not suppress symptoms, but instead address 'deeper causes.' Thus, drugs would interfere with the 'real treatment,' that is, psychotherapy.

By the time I entered residency, all psychotic patients were receiving drugs. Even so, for psychoanalysts in charge of in-patient units, these agents were only a means of behavioural control, calming patients suffi-

ciently to make them accessible to what the analysts saw as more definitive treatment.

While treating psychotic patients humanistically is laudable in principle, failure to recognize the gravity of an illness can lead to negative
consequences. In one case treated at the hospital where I was training as
a resident, two young schizophrenics became physically involved while
on the ward. Instead of being separated, they were treated with couple
therapy; this procedure was written up and duly appeared in the *Canadian Journal of Psychiatry*.[45] Although the article provided no follow-up
on the patients, it managed to imply that the intervention had somehow
been successful. (Later in the book I will discuss how the absence of follow-up has consistently led to misjudgments about the effectiveness of
psychotherapy.) In fact, both of the patients described in this case
report did poorly, and both required a course of ECT after the therapy.
Neither of them ever returned to school or held a job. (One committed
suicide five years later.) Although by the time of the publication I was
already on faculty, I felt outraged at this misrepresentation of the facts,
and I wrote a letter to the editor that suggested the case might have
been mismanaged. However, I did not volunteer that I had seen the
disaster unfolding with my own eyes. I expected Henry Kravitz, one of
the co-authors of the paper, to be angry, but he surprised me with a
benevolent response, saying, 'You should have said you were there – you
don't have to be Alexander Solzhenitsyn.'

Resistance to physical and drug treatment of schizophrenic patients
ended in the late 1960s. Phillip May, a psychiatrist at UCLA, published a
study that was impossible to refute.[46] Schizophrenic patients admitted to
hospital were randomly assigned to medication alone, ECT alone, psychotherapy alone, or a combination of these treatments. The most useful therapy, by far, turned out to be medication, and psychotherapy
failed to add to its effectiveness.

To his credit, Henry Kravitz read May's book a few years after it was
published, and accepted these findings. After that, the wards at his hospital stopped offering intensive psychotherapy and long-term admissions for schizophrenia. Kravitz spent the next thirty years of his life
advocating analytic therapy – but only for non-psychotic patients.

Psychoanalysis and Its Claims to Cure

Lengthy admissions focusing on psychotherapeutic treatment for serious
mental illness were common in American psychiatry until the 1980s. Hos-

pital units of this kind were developed in major teaching hospitals at universities such as Harvard, Yale, and Columbia. Others were located at private hospitals with weaker links to medical research. The Menninger Clinic in Kansas, Chestnut Lodge in Maryland, and the Austen Riggs Center in the Berkshires were all independent of academia, maintaining only tenuous connections to nearby universities. They attracted limited numbers of wealthy patients looking for a 'talking cure,' who were willing to sacrifice significant income to obtain the 'best' form of therapy. These hospitals offered long-term hospital admissions in which the primary form of treatment was psychoanalytic therapy.

Today the market for this type of treatment has virtually dried up. Insurance doesn't pay for it, and few families have a strong enough belief in it to pay out of pocket. As a result, private, analytically oriented hospitals have withered on the vine. The Menninger Hospital in Topeka, once dominant in American psychiatric education, has closed. Chestnut Lodge, after a period of offering brief admissions and rehabilitation for psychotic patients, went bankrupt and also shut down. The exception is Austen Riggs, a small hospital that remains in relatively healthy shape by focusing on a boutique market. (Even at Riggs, patients rarely stay in the hospital for long.)

The misadventures of psychoanalysis in trying to cure psychosis illustrate an important factor behind its decline. Many psychiatrists who trained during the heyday of analysis believed they were learning a complex method that could cure otherwise incurable patients. When that expectation failed, they became more conservative about whom to accept for treatment. A few were disillusioned enough to abandon analysis entirely. Other analysts remain proud of a training that helped them to understand people. John Gunderson, a Harvard professor who is an expert on borderline personality disorder, and who still uses analytic methods in his clinical practice, told me that psychoanalysis failed to deliver on its larger promises, and that the bottom line was that sicker patients did not improve with treatment.[47]

Today, everyone agrees that drugs are effective, and that analytic therapy is not helpful when patients are acutely psychotic. Still, schizophrenia is a chronic disease that can last a lifetime. Might it still be possible for analytic treatment to help patients recover once acute episodes subside? While Gunderson was at the National Institutes of Mental Health in the early 1970s he conducted a study of the effectiveness of long-term psychoanalytic therapy in schizophrenia.[48] The results found no advantage for an analytic approach over purely supportive therapy. Following schizophrenic patients closely offers them a relationship that can help them to cope, and makes it more likely that they will comply with medication. But analytic therapy does not make a difference in the long-term outcome.

These results accord with the findings of Tom McGlashan, who followed up a large number of patients treated at Chestnut Lodge.[49] After years of intensive analytic therapy, schizophrenic patients treated at the Lodge and receiving intensive analytic follow-up did no better than those treated with less arduous and expensive forms of therapy. At best, careful and close follow-up of these patients is a useful adjunct to pharmacotherapy. The only evidence that talking therapies have something to add to drug treatment comes from studies with 'sociotherapy' (i.e., rehabilitation programs),[50] and the use of cognitive behavioural therapy.[51]

John Gunderson told me he had to conclude, somewhat painfully, that the heroes of his past had proved to be flawed, and that their claims to cure psychosis had been arrogant. He noted that very few of those who advocated and wrote about psychotherapy in schizophrenia had actually carried out these treatments on more than a few selected patients. Analysts taught residents in hospitals how to treat psychotic patients, but when they went to their own offices they saw only neurotic patients. The gurus of analytic treatment for schizophrenia were advocating a method that they themselves were unwilling to put into practice.

Gunderson now believes that psychoanalysis, as a method of treatment, is useful for only a small fraction of the clinical population that psychiatrists see. But the deeper problem he sees is the way analysts draw vast conclusions based on clinical experience alone. In Gunderson's view, 'the analytic community failed to understand the nature of scientific evidence.'

To be fair, other medical specialties have had similar problems. Still, most have always been committed, at least in principle, to empiricism, and practice has gradually become more evidence-based over time. Yet the failure of analysis as a treatment for psychosis can be seen in a broader context.

Even more tellingly, psychoanalysis has failed to demonstrate its usefulness for the neurotic problems studied by Freud. (I will return to this issue in chapter 5.) Several of the academics I interviewed emphasized this point. Donald Klein, a research psychiatrist at Columbia, told me that psychoanalysis went into decline when it could not even demonstrate efficacy for common problems such as anxiety and depression. Klein also noted that one of the few long-term follow-up studies, on patients treated at the Menninger Clinic,[52] showed surprisingly poor results. Another informant, Leston Havens, a well-known Harvard psychiatrist, resigned from the Boston Psychoanalytic Society when he concluded that analysis lacked proof of its efficacy and showed no interest in obtaining it. Efforts by the American Psychoanalytic Association to design a large-scale study of treatment efficacy had ended in a fiasco: the results were so unimpressive that the Association suppressed them. Most of the data were never published; only a few, largely negative findings remained buried in an obscure report. (The detailed sequence of events in this story is described in Shorter's *History of Psychiatry*).

Psychiatric Journals and Textbooks

While the *American Journal of Psychiatry* is the most widely read publication in the field, it ranks second in prestige to the *Archives of General Psychiatry*. The *Archives* published its first issue in July 1959. The new journal had split off from an earlier AMA publication, the *Archives of Neurology and Psychiatry*, at a point when psychiatry had finally earned full independence from neurology. Its editor, Roy Grinker, was the psychoanalyst who had studied war neuroses and who retained a deep interest in research.

In his opening editorial, Grinker announced his vision: 'We shall publish contributions from all disciplines, whether morphological, physiological, biochemical, endocrinological, psychosomatic, psychological, psychiatric, child-psychiatric, psychoanalytical, sociological or anthropological, that are related to the study of the behavior of Man in health and illness.'[53] Under Grinker the *Archives* did indeed publish a wide range of papers. (Nonetheless, the journal began as a product of its times: the first article in the first issue was an 'opinion piece' by the Chicago analyst John Gedo entitled 'Some Difficulties of Psychotherapeutic Practice.')[54]

Under Grinker, the *Archives* was always lively, but after his retirement in 1970 the journal's complexion changed. In chapter 6 I will discuss the work of the second editor, Daniel Xavier Freedman, a former analyst turned biological researcher. Under Freedman, the 'impact factor' of the journal (i.e., how often its articles are quoted by others) went up remarkably, and today is more than twice that of the *American Journal*. The only way to publish in the *Archives* is to present hard data backed up by statistics. One almost never sees a case history in its pages. As psychiatry became more biological, so did the *Archives*, leading one wag to refer to it as the 'Journal of Body Fluids.' By and large, researchers read the journal, and practitioners do not. Still, its impact factor reflects a very strong influence on academic psychiatry.

The *American Journal of Psychiatry* was a little slower to change. During the 1950s and 1960s, Francis Braceland, a psychiatrist working in a private hospital in Connecticut was the editor; in his time more articles influenced by psychoanalysis appeared. Then in 1970 John Nemiah, a well-known Boston psychoanalyst, took over. While Nemiah had a strong analytic commitment, he was willing to move with the times. Over the twenty-four years of his stewardship, the *American Journal* gradually evolved into a scientific forum, with less and less clinical opinion.

In 1994, Nancy Andreasen of the University of Iowa became editor of the *American Journal*. Andreasen is a former literature professor who became a psychiatrist and a researcher. (A convert can sometimes be 'holier than the pope.') Under her leadership, the *Journal* publishes very little about psychoanalysis (with the exception of book reviews), but a great deal about biological research.

Textbooks provide another measure of the changes in academic psychiatry. In 1967, two eclectic analysts, Alfred Freedman and Harold Kaplan, published the *Comprehensive Textbook of Psychiatry*.[55] The first edition was a real milestone. When the text came out, I read it cover to cover, then bought several of the subsequent editions. Freedman retired in the 1970s, and was replaced by Kaplan, a hard-working man who gave the rest of his life to the book. The many editions he edited became the standard text for American psychiatry. Even after Kaplan died, to be replaced by Benjamin and Virginia Sadock, the 9th edition, published in 1998,[56] is still referred to by almost everyone as 'Kaplan.'

While both Freedman and Kaplan were analysts, they had a much broader agenda, and tried to make their book truly comprehensive, addressing every aspect of psychiatry. Heinz Lehmann authored two superb chapters in the first edition, describing the clinical features of schizophrenia and mood disorders. While psychoanalysis and its theories figured prominently in the early editions of Kaplan, and some original chapters have been kept in the latest one, these sections, which have changed little over the years, now seem historical. In contrast, the rest of Kaplan has changed so much as to be unrecognizable. The vast expansion of the text (now in two large volumes) is mainly the result of advances in biological research.

Looking Backward

In the nineteenth century, psychiatry, rooted in state hospitals and asylums, separated from general medicine. The development of academic psychiatry in university-affiliated general hospitals was an attempt to overcome this barrier. Ironically, the dominance of analytic theories in these new settings only created a new and different gap between medicine and psychiatry.

Academic psychiatry, as long as it was dominated by psychoanalysis, produced very little research. In the 1960s many of the top American medical schools provided clinical services focused on analytic therapy. Yet little or no effort was made to determine the effectiveness of these treatments. It is not surprising, therefore, that psychiatry lost respect. As we will see later in this book, psychiatry only regained its position within medicine when it found new theoretical roots in the neurosciences, and began to base its treatment methods on evidence.

chapter 2

Three Famous Universities

To illustrate the relationship between psychoanalysis and academic psychiatry, this chapter will draw on three 'case examples' from American universities: Harvard, Johns Hopkins, and Columbia. These famous medical schools have set the trajectory for psychiatry in both the United States and Canada. Each of these departments has had a unique history. At Harvard, psychoanalysis became dominant. Hopkins became a 'leader of the opposition' to analysis. Columbia attempted to find a middle ground.

Harvard: Where Analysis Once Reigned

Harvard University's name has always held magic. In medicine, its professors have authored standard texts, defining the direction of entire specialties. When psychoanalysts took leading positions at Harvard in the 1950s, the movement could claim a major victory.

Harvard is unique in never having had, even on paper, a single department of psychiatry. One might say that it is not a kingdom, but a loose federation of duchies. Each hospital runs its own affairs, and supports a separate residency training program. The system was only loosely governed by a 'combined executive.'

The radically decentralized Harvard system allowed hospitals to offer highly specialized programs. Its residency training programs did not provide broad experience in all areas of psychiatry, and they were narrowly based. Fifty years ago, at several Harvard-affiliated hospitals, the focus was almost entirely on psychoanalytic psychotherapy.

Surprisingly, the most influential site for psychiatric training at Harvard at that time was a state hospital. The Boston Psychopathic Hospital, later renamed the Massachusetts Mental Health Center, is not far from downtown. Its close affiliation to Harvard made 'Mass Mental' atypical. In the 1950s, Jack Ewalt, a Group member for the Advancement of Psychiatry and community psychiatrist, was the chief, but training at Mass Mental was dominated by a psychoanalyst.

The Charisma of Elvin Semrad

Elvin Semrad is an important character in the history of the relationship between psychoanalysis and academic psychiatry. A grandfatherly and portly man with a white beard, Semrad is described by many of his students as resembling Santa Claus. Semrad was devoted to his patients. He worked well into the evening and on weekends, rarely taking vacations, and did not seem to have much of an outside life. He had enormous charisma, and his unforgettable teaching style influenced a whole generation of students. Paul Soloff, a Pittsburgh psychopharmacology researcher who does not practise analytic therapy, still remembers him with awe and respect.

For Elvin Semrad, the key to treating patients was to sit and listen. One psychiatrist in personal therapy with Semrad described him to me as a 'silent analyst.' But with his students, Semrad could be voluble and pithy. They even collected and published a series of his most quotable aphorisms.[1] A psychiatrist on Semrad's couch heard of this project and asked him why he was so unresponsive to *him*. (The analyst's answer, as usual, was silence.)

Semrad believed that schizophrenia was nothing but a response to a faulty environment. His view was that everyone is a little crazy – psychotic patients being just a little more so. However controversial his ideas about schizophrenia, Semrad had great empathy for those who suffered from the disease. Several of his students told me that patients could describe to Semrad, much more clearly than to anyone else, what it *felt* like to be psychotic. Leston Havens, a psychiatrist who studied under Semrad, describes him as 'an existentialist behind an analytic facade.'[2]

Paul McHugh, a professor at Johns Hopkins, emphasizes that the problem with Semrad was that he assumed that these inner experiences were the *cause* of the illness, rather than the other way round.[3] Actually, none of the psychiatrists I spoke to about Semrad still believes in a psychological theory of psychosis. They now see their old teacher as sincere but misguided. Semrad had entirely dismissed all biological theories of schizophrenia, and was firmly against the use of drugs, which he thought undercut the more 'important' work of psychotherapy. Needless to say, this approach was totally impractical, particularly in a state hospital. As one of his students told me, Jack Ewalt would quietly tell the residents: 'Go ahead and prescribe, just don't tell Semrad.'

Ironically, Semrad had very little personal experience treating schizophrenic patients. He had seen cases early in his career, but his own clinical practice consisted almost entirely of patients in formal psychoanalysis. After devoting hours to teaching on psychotic patients, Semrad would go to his office to conduct training analyses or to treat wealthy patients who were not severely ill. This discrepancy between the two tiers of psychiatric treatment was pervasive. Hardly anyone admitted to a state hospital could have afforded the fees of a psychoanalyst.

The situation in Canada was much the same. When I trained in psychiatry at McGill, our analytically oriented teachers taught us to talk to psychotic patients on the wards, but rarely took them into their own practices. When they did try to treat psychosis with talking therapy, the results were unimpressive (and sometimes disastrous).

As with other charismatic therapists of his epoch, Semrad's specialty was the demonstration interview. This was the perfect opportunity for a masterful performance by a senior clinician. One could vastly impress students with empathy and acumen after spending an hour with a patient. I saw many of these interviews over the years, carried out by local celebrities or visiting professors. They reflected a time when clinical charisma was more important than knowledge. Today, large audiences are more likely to show up for data-driven talks in Power Point.

Demonstration interviews provided a great show for the audience. Watching experts at work was often entertaining, and occasionally illuminating. Unfortunately, patients rarely benefited from these encounters. (In one memorable episode at McGill, a patient committed suicide after being interviewed by an inquiring but unempathic visiting analyst, after which demonstration interviews were barred for years.)

Elvin Semrad, in spite of the influence he had in his own time, has been gradually forgotten. One reason is that he worked in an oral culture, and wrote almost nothing. Another is that his ideas were never supported by data. Semrad was a guru, but most young psychiatrists today would not even recognize his name.

The psychoanalytic treatment of schizophrenia has also been discarded. As discussed in chapter 1, research has not supported its efficacy. Mass Mental's current mission would also be unrecognizable to Semrad.

The hospital no longer admits patients, but has become a centre for community psychiatry and the rehabilitation of chronic patients, and a major site for biological research into the causes of psychotic illness.

The Harvard Network

In the 1950s, the Massachusetts Mental Health Center's training program seeded all the other hospitals in the Harvard network. Psychiatrists who had trained under Semrad became clinical leaders and teachers.

Cambridge Hospital, located close to the main university campus, has traditionally been a centre for psychotherapy. John Mack, an analyst known for a Pulitzer Prize–winning biography of T.E. Lawrence,[4] was the hospital chief at Cambridge for many years. (Later, to the embarassment of his Harvard colleagues, Mack wrote a book supporting the reality of alien abduction by extraterrestrials.[5])

Beth Israel Hospital also has a strong psychotherapy tradition. Located near downtown Boston, it was built by the Jewish community, traditional allies of psychoanalysis. The founder of its psychiatry department was Grete Bibring, one of Freud's students. Bibring, a woman of culture and charm, represented psychoanalysis in its original Viennese incarnation. John Nemiah, long-time editor of the *American Journal of Psychiatry*, succeeded her. Nemiah wanted to bring analysis into the psychiatric mainstream, and hired a psychoanalyst, Peter Sifneos, who carried out research on short-term analytic therapy that attracted interest in the 1970s.[6]

The central hospital for teaching and research at Harvard Medical School is the Massachusetts General Hospital. Its psychiatry department naturally developed closer relationships to other medical specialities. These links were associated with a weakening of the influence of psychoanalysis. In the 1950s, the chief of psychiatry at Massachusetts General was Eric Lindemann. A noted psychoanalyst, Lindemann is still remembered for his clinical study of survivors of a famous nightclub fire in Boston.[7] But Lindemann was out of touch with the needs of the hospital. When he retired, a petition was circulated among the medical staff urging the search committee not to appoint another psychoanalyst.[8]

Physicians in general hospitals often need psychiatric consultations for their patients. In the heyday of analysis, these consults were often considered useless. The general complaint was that consultants offered complex theoretical formulations but provided little practical advice.

Thus, psychiatric input drew little or no respect from the medical community. When I interned at a teaching hospital in Montreal in the mid-1960s, I would hear physicians say: 'Psychiatrists always have an opinion about what's wrong but never tell you what to do about it.'

In 1967, Massachusetts General recruited Leon Eisenberg, a professor from Johns Hopkins, to replace Lindemann. At the time, Eisenberg was the only university professor and hospital chief at Harvard who was *not* a psychoanalyst. Although he faced major opposition from analytic faculty members, Eisenberg was ahead of his time. He has written vivid descriptions of being almost the only person in his academic milieu to question the psychoanalytic approach to psychiatry.[9] Yet what was radical then is mainstream now. Eisenberg's empirical outlook helped to make Massachusetts General a leading centre for psychiatric research at Harvard, which it still is.

McLean Hospital may be the most famous site in the Harvard psychiatry network.[10] A private mental hospital built in the late nineteenth century, it is located in the suburb of Belmont, far from Harvard Square or Boston, on beautiful grounds planned by the famous landscape designer Frederick Olmstead. McLean was never a purely analytic setting, and it always promoted research. Yet, like other private hospitals, McLean catered to the wealthy, specializing in long admissions designed to promote extensive psychotherapy. Even today, McLean runs a rather fancy private ward called 'The Pavilion,' glossily advertised in the *New Yorker* magazine.

McLean has evolved greatly in recent decades. In the 1970s, Shervert Frazier, a Texan who had headed the National Institutes of Mental Health, came to McLean as chief. Frazier told me he found the hospital $8 million in debt, largely due to a restriction on the type of patients it accepted. Frazier described McLean's complex process to determine suitability for psychotherapy, which involved multiple interviews and case conferences: 'It was more difficult to get into McLean than to get into Harvard. This was a graduate center, and you had to be qualified. Getting accepted for treatment was an ordeal.'[11]

These complex admission procedures had developed in a period when McLean almost never admitted psychotic patients. Most clients were wealthy and young, and many suffered from personality disorders, conditions that produce aberrant behaviour rather than classical psychiatric symptoms. These patients (or more often their parents) demanded in-patient care, and McLean could afford to be selective.

When more seriously ill cases were admitted, they were often well-known people from the Boston area. Robert Lowell, who suffered from bipolar illness for most of his life, wrote a poem about his time at McLean.[12] Sylvia Plath was admitted after a serious suicide attempt, and described McLean colourfully in her famous novel *The Bell Jar*.[13] More recently, the hospital has been colourfully portrayed in two books (later made into films), *Girl Interrupted* and *A Beautiful Mind*.[14]

By the time Frazier arrived, the market for lengthy admissions had dried up. By accepting short-term admissions of sicker patients, Frazier rapidly filled up beds and erased the deficit. He also accepted adolescents, who, he said, 'helped keep up volume, even though they just about tore the place up.'[15] Frazier also put McLean on the map in biological research. He raised millions for new laboratories, recruiting prominent researchers in schizophrenia, such as Seymour Kety, who conducted pioneering genetic studies of psychosis,[16] and Phillip Holtzman, who identified abnormal eye movements as a marker for schizophrenia.[17]

At first, psychoanalysts on the executive committee of McLean balked at all these changes, asking, 'What do these new people know about dynamic psychiatry?'[18] But the old guard was consistently outvoted. The hospital board, dominated by Boston Brahmins, was concerned about the bottom line, and was happy with Frazier's administration.

Shervert Frazier sees himself as a man who has always wanted to bring people together. Although originally trained as an analyst, he moved into a research career. Frazier still believes analysis has its place in psychiatric practice and education. His view of his leadership at McLean is that he was adding, not subtracting.

These changes took place in the 1970s, marking a watershed in the role of psychoanalysis at Harvard. The peak of its influence had already passed. By the end of the century, Health Maintenance Organizations had effectively eliminated long-term admissions. For a while, some American hospitals (like McLean) actually went to Canada to recruit patients (the Ontario government had a generous policy paying for stays in the USA). In the end, however, beds had to be closed, and the mission of the hospital had to change.

McLean Hospital is still struggling to keep afloat in the new climate, and half of its grounds have been sold off to pay the bills. Still, McLean has successfully moved with the times. It is well known for the quality of its research. Many of the new generation of leaders there are biologically oriented psychiatrists.

Johns Hopkins: A Department Ahead of Its Time

When Johns Hopkins University opened a medical school in the 1890s, it was designed to be 'state of the art.' The Hopkins model greatly influenced medical education. One of its faculty members, Abraham Flexner, wrote a report[19] that led to higher standards for training physicians all over the United States. (Flexner also surveyed all the medical faculties in Canada.)

Johns Hopkins became the first centre for what today is termed evidence-based medicine. And Hopkins has retained its prestige, right into the twenty-first century. The most famous physician ever to work there was William Osler. A Canadian by birth, Osler started at McGill, moved to Philadelphia, and ended his career at Oxford. But he spent his greatest years in Baltimore. At Hopkins, Osler wrote a famous textbook, *The Principles and Practice of Medicine*, the standard and authoritative text for a generation of medical graduates.[20] In his time, Osler knew almost everything there was to be known, and even included a few pages discussing the recently published theories of Sigmund Freud.

Osler was also important because of his ideas about medical education. In the nineteenth century medicine was divided into a set of 'schools,' each built around a particular therapeutic method and a charismatic leader, the very situation that has plagued psychiatry. Osler replaced 'schools' with a unified scientific model built around detailed study and the observation of patients.

Paul McHugh, a long-time chair at Hopkins, describes psychiatry as being 'pre-Oslerian.'[21] What he means is that its division into various schools of psychotherapy (and pharmacology) still reflects a weak commitment to empiricism and the lack of a unifying model. The picture drawn by McHugh seems to parallel Thomas Kuhn's 'pre-paradigmatic' stage in the history of science.[22] One reason why the Hopkins psychiatry department was never dominated by psychoanalysis was probably the continuing influence of Osler.

The unique history of Hopkins was shaped by another great psychiatrist. For thirty-two years, from 1909 to 1941, the department was under the leadership of Adolf Meyer,[23] a Swiss immigrant recruited from Columbia. Like Elvin Semrad, Meyer was a great teacher who wrote little, and whose thoughts were only put into print by his students after his death. Yet Meyer's ideas had a much more profound and continuing influence on academic psychiatry. Many of his students became departmental chairs. The American Psychiatric Association still sponsors an

Adolf Meyer Lecture, a major theoretical review presented at its annual meeting.

Meyer termed his point of view 'psychobiology,'[24] by which he meant that mental illnesses are reactions to stress, modulated by predispositions. But Meyer, like almost everyone else in American psychiatry at that time, emphasized the role of the environment. He was also largely responsible for the detailed history and 'mental status' that are now standard in all psychiatric assessments. He encouraged the development of epidemiological research and follow-up studies to determine whether patients benefit from treatment. Finally, Meyer believed in practical treatment methods and prevention through 'mental hygiene.' He believed that psychotherapy was necessary for most patients, but denied that it had to take the form set out by Freud.

After the Second World War, Meyer's ideas became increasingly marginal. Shortly before his death, he wrote despairingly in his diary that everything he had ever worked for seemed to be collapsing.[25] But the old professor was altogether too pessimistic. The Hopkins tradition was intact, and it strongly shaped the ideas of his successors.

John Whitehorn served as chair at Hopkins from 1941 to 1960. Although Whitehorn had started his career as a biochemical researcher, he devoted his time at Hopkins almost exclusively to psychotherapy research. Whitehorn produced data suggesting that the personal qualities of therapists are more important than their techniques.[26] Research on psychotherapy was important for a field that had previously been the subject of clinical lore and speculation alone. In 1952, the British psychologist Hans Eysenck had pointed out the lack of empirical evidence for the efficacy of almost any form of psychotherapy.[27] This was a challenge that had to be answered.

Jerome Frank, one of the great pioneers of psychotherapy research, spent his professional life at Hopkins.[28] Frank was a psychiatrist with a PhD in psychology and a strong commitment to research findings. His famous book *Persuasion and Healing* was first published in 1962.[29] It had, and still has, a great influence on how psychiatrists view psychotherapy. Taking his cue from Meyer, Frank provided a model that explains why, independent of its theory, psychoanalysis can sometimes work, and why other, less arduous methods, based on different theories, work equally well.

Frank saw psychotherapy as a process of remoralization. Patients come to therapy demoralized, and improve by regaining hope. Thus, the process, as opposed to the content, of treatment is most crucial to recovery. The main engine of recovery in psychotherapy is not technique but a healing relationship. Thus, talking about childhood or past events may not be a crucial factor in therapy. It may not matter what theory therapists believe in, as long as patients are willing to accept it.

Contemporary ideas about psychotherapy have come to correspond rather closely to what Frank wrote about forty years ago. As will be discussed later in this book, a large body of research findings has emerged to show that technique plays a lesser role in the efficacy of therapy than the quality of the doctor–patient relationship.[30] Moreover, there is little reason to believe that any particular form of treatment is more effective than any other. The explanation is that common, or 'non-specific' factors, most particularly the quality of the therapeutic relationship, are the most important predictors of results. Obviously, these findings shed doubt on the unique efficacy of psychoanalysis.

A child psychiatrist Leo Kanner (1895–1981) was another great professor at Hopkins. Kanner stood firmly in the tradition of eclecticism, never accepting the claims of his analyst colleagues to cure mental illness. But even Kanner could not help being influenced by the climate of his times, which led him to make a famous mistake.

Kanner had been the first psychiatrist to describe early infantile autism.[31] He was unclear as to whether the syndrome he described was genetic, environmental, or both. Kanner, observing relationships between these children and their parents, coined the term 'refrigerator mother' to describe a lack of bonding to an autistic child. This concept was interpreted as implying that unresponsive mothers could be responsible for unresponsive children. Later in life, Kanner was sorry for what he had said, and wrote an apologetic book that defended the role of parents.[32]

But Kanner's error haunted child psychiatry for decades to come. Chicago psychoanalyst Bruno Bettelheim wrote a book called *The Empty Fortress*, accusing mothers of causing autism through emotional rejection.[33] Bettelheim's ideas had tragic consequences, for both mothers and children. (Bettelheim, a cultural hero of the 1960s, was discredited after his death when it was discovered he had lied about his qualifications, faked data, and physically assaulted children attending his 'Orthogenic School' for troubled children.)[34]

Today we know that autism is a brain disease with a strong heritable component, for which parents are in no way responsible.[35] Kanner's 'refrigerator mothers' were simply reacting to children who were incapable of emotional contact. Seeing effects as causes has led to many errors in psychiatry.

Hopkins continues to be, as it always has been, a centre for empiricism and rigour. Thus, the name of the department was changed to Psychiatry and Behavioral Sciences when Joel Elkes, a pioneer of psychopharmacology, was chair (1965–73). His successor Paul McHugh (1975–2001) became well known as a critic of psychoanalysis, as well as of one of its offshoots, the 'recovered memory' movement.

Columbia: A Happy Medium?

New York has always been and still is the epicentre of American psychoanalysis. The New York Psychoanalytic Society was founded in 1911, early in the history of the movement.[36] Yet for another twenty years psychoanalytic training required a trip to Europe. Then Abraham Brill, the first translator of Freud's books into English, founded the New York Psychoanalytic Institute, the first in the United States.

After Hitler came to power, many prominent European analysts, all of whom had trained with Freud or with his disciples, moved to New York. The list included Heinz Hartmann, who developed a modified model of psychoanalysis called 'ego psychology';[37] Margaret Mahler, who developed theories about the role of separation and individuation in early childhood;[38] Kurt Eissler, later in charge of the Freud Archives;[39] and Paul Federn, who pioneered the psychotherapy of schizophrenia.[40]

Due to its close links to Freud and his students, the New York Psychoanalytic Institute became famous for its orthodoxy. Its leaders, never closely linked to a university, were intensely proud of their fealty to analytic tradition. The New York Institute was also famous for expelling dissidents who dared to develop their own versions of the Freudian model. Among these were Karen Horney (who, apocryphally, claimed to have marched out of the Institute defiantly singing a spiritual about freedom).[41] This was also the time when Erich Fromm was excluded from the International Psychoanalytic Association, and forced to open his own institute in Mexico City.[42]

Sandor Rado, a colourful Hungarian described by Donald Klein (see below) as 'a little bull of a man,' was a dissident who never officially broke with mainstream analysis, even though he rejected many traditional ideas and openly mocked Freud's formulations. Rado's own theory, which he called 'adaptational psychodynamics' was an early attempt to fuse analysis and behaviourism.[43] One of Rado's collaborators, Abram Kardiner (who published a book about his own analysis with Freud),[44] was an eclectic who developed links between psychoanalysis and cultural anthropology.

Rado and Kardiner left the New York Institute in 1945, largely because of its conservatism. They founded an new Institute of Psychoanalytic Medicine, which was planned to be both physically and conceptually within a university hospital at Columbia. The Center for Psychoanalysis, as it is now called, remains somewhat exceptional in American academic psychiatry. There is one other institute in New York affiliated with a psychiatry department, initially at Downstate, and later located at New York University. Emory University in Atlanta and the University of Colorado have parallel arrangements.

Columbia was the perfect place to bring analysis into mainstream psychiatry. It had unique resources, in that its main teaching centre, the New York State Psychiatric Institute, is a psychiatric hospital with a stable budget provided by the state, treating all classes of patients with mental illness. (The University of Pittsburgh and UCLA have a similar relationship to their state governments, and both departments have long been leaders in academic psychiatry.) The Institute has had a distinguished history, starting with Adolf Meyer, who was its chief before he went to Hopkins. The institute has always attracted, and continues to attract, large amounts of research dollars.

A psychoanalyst, Laurence Kolb, was chair at Columbia from 1954 to 1975. When he retired, the medical school decided it was time for a change. Edward Sachar, trained as an analyst, had become noted for his research on the neuroendocrinology of mental illness.[45] Under his leadership, Columbia moved resources into basic research and clinical investigation.

Sachar recruited Donald Klein to be director of research. Klein has long been, and continues to be, a gadfly for psychiatry. Well known for his research on psychopharmacology and anxiety disorders,[46] Klein has been a major force at Columbia and a consistent opponent of analysis. Yet in the 1950s Klein had been a trainee at the New York Psychoanalytic Institute. Like many young psychiatrists of his era, he saw analysis as being at the cutting edge of psychiatry. Never a man to accept orthodoxy, however, Klein left the institute without completing his training.

When Sachar was unable to work because of a stroke, he was replaced by Herbert Pardes, a former director of the National Institutes of Mental Health, who remained as chair at Columbia from 1984 to 2000.

Under his leadership, the department moved more sharply into a research and biological mode. These were glory days for Columbia.[47] Eric Kandel, who became the second psychiatrist in history to win a Nobel Prize in 2000, became the leader of basic research. Columbia recruited high-impact clinical researchers studying the neurobiology of mental disorders, and also became one of the predominant sites in the world for psychiatric epidemiology. Pardes even convinced New York State to construct an entirely new Psychiatric Institute, a building that now stands proudly overlooking the Hudson River.

Otto Kernberg, a famous analyst trained at the Menninger Clinic, had been recruited to Columbia in the early 1970s. But Kernberg was forced out by the new departmental priorities, and left for Cornell, where he still works. Even after this departure, the Institute continued to run a psychoanalytically oriented in-patient ward. Under the psychoanalyst Michael Stone the unit mainly admitted young people with behavioural problems and personality disorders. While the clientele closely resembled that of private hospitals such as McLean, the State of New York was willing to pay for their treatment.

The psychoanalytic institute at Columbia remains physically and administratively part of the psychiatry department. Although it does not produce research, it has a continuing influence at Columbia. Even today, most residents applying to the psychiatry department want to be therapists. Klein complains that he was unable to change the selection criteria for the program to attract researchers. As is the case in many departments of psychiatry, analysts remain in demand as teachers.

Columbia has also bucked the general trend in which young psychiatrists have stopped applying to analytic institutes. In most centres, being an analyst no longer carries prestige, and does not help one's career. In New York, however, one can still earn a living practising psychoanalysis. Residents at Columbia also like its analytic training because of the eclectic curriculum. Students are no longer expected to read the complete works of Sigmund Freud, a requirement that has long been a standard rite of passage for candidates everywhere else in the psychoanalytic world. Moreover, unlike the New York Psychoanalytic Institute, the Columbia Institute does not expect its graduates to commit themselves totally to analytic practice.

Has Columbia therefore found a happy medium between the domination and exclusion of psychoanalysis in academic psychiatry? In the eyes of Donald Klein, 'the Center for Psychoanalysis isn't doing much.'[48] What Klein means is that this group fails to meet standards normally expected of any academic group provided space and funding at a medical school. While Columbia has provided an enclave for teaching a specific therapeutic technique, its analysts taught but did not publish empirical research in medical journals.

Psychoanalysis has always been an art, and not a science. Freud, a product of his times, was sceptical about empirical methods as a way of assessing the results of analysis. Yet today, every form of treatment is expected to be supported by research data. Studies to determine the efficacy of analytic therapy are badly needed.

The psychoanalytic movement has responded weakly and grudgingly to these challenges. Otto Kernberg, when president of the International Psychoanalytic Association, created a fund for psychoanalytic research. But its limited resources have been insufficient to meet a large number of requests for funding. When questions arise about controversial and expensive treatment modalities, academic medicine has to take the lead in conducting systematic testing. A centre for psychoanalysis at a great medical school should carry out research. This has not been the case at Columbia. Paul McHugh of Hopkins believes that, in the long run, analysis will entirely disappear from academic psychiatry.[49] Creating psychoanalytic institutes inside university departments has not made this outcome any less likely.

chapter 3

The Inner World of Psychoanalysis

Institutes and Isolation

The academic world promotes freedom of inquiry. At the same time, academia has established standards for the acceptance of new knowledge. Data and ideas are accountable, that is, judged through 'peer review' by experts who can evaluate the evidence. For this reason, universities are the best place to test psychological theories, and the best place to determine whether therapeutic methods are effective.

If psychoanalysis is, as it claims, a science of human behaviour, and an established method of treating mental illness, why is it not offered as a form of advanced training in medical or graduate schools? The answer lies in history.

Freud's creation of institutes, separate from academia, was a reaction to the rejection of his movement by mainstream European psychiatry.[1] At that time, it was unlikely that universities would devote significant resources to a maverick discipline. Instead, the institutes took on the task of training new recruits in analytic theory and methods. After graduation, practitioners joined psychoanalytic societies that were fully independent of universities.

When analysis came to the United States, it established its own institutes. In 1931, the New York Psychoanalytic Institute had recruited a Berlin analyst, Sandor Rado, to set up its training program. (As noted in chapter 2, Rado later became dissatisfied with orthodoxy, and left to create a separate institute at Columbia University.) Elsewhere in America, newly created institutes were also founded by recruits from Europe. Franz Alexander, one of the most creative early analysts, was brought to Chicago to found its institute. Another German analyst, Ernst Simmel, founded the institute in Los Angeles. After Hitler came to power, Jewish analysts had to leave Germany. Since psychoanalysis was actively suppressed in Germany, non-Jewish analysts such as Karen Horney were also forced to emigrate. Once Austria was taken over in 1938, Freud and his daughter Anna moved to England. America became a new home for the psychoanalytic movement. Many prominent figures from Vienna became training analysts at the New York Psychoanalytic. Staffed by Freud's students and colleagues, this institute remained a bastion of orthodoxy for decades for come.

The result was that psychoanalysis was taught only in institutes, not in psychiatry programs. Many residencies did not even have psychotherapy in their curricula. One might have thought this situation would have changed once analysis gained influence in academic psychiatry. Yet even then, institutes remained separate. They provided an inner sanctum where an elite group of training analysts controlled education, and where society members met weekly for case presentations and theoretical discussions.

The story of analytic institutes in America has been beautifully told by Douglas Kirsner in his book *Unfree Associations*.[2] In many cities, divisions within the movement led to the creation of multiple and competing institutes. Some dissidents disagreed over theoretical issues. In many cases, however, the splits were almost entirely the result of power struggles over which faculty member could gain the desired status of training analyst.

In New York, a few dissenters moved into universities, while others formed separate institutes. The situation was similar in Boston, where a series of splits led to the creation of three institutes: one traditional and orthodox, one 'modern' and eclectic, and one specifically designed for psychologists. A split between competing analysts also led to Los Angeles having two institutes. (Montreal also has two institutes, but as with so many other institutions in that city, one is English and one French.)

The outcome of this process was the isolation of the analytic movement from the academic world. Ultimately, this created an anachronistic situation. Psychoanalytic institutes were mainly interested in training a new generation to carry on tradition. They paid lip service to progress, but rarely supported research. In contrast to universities, institutes were not in a position to revise theories or develop new ways of practice. As Kirsner points out, analysis cannot claim to be maintaining its own 'scientific' standards if it does not function as a science. Ultimately, the isolation of institutes from academia has been a major factor in the downfall of the movement. To understand why, we need to explore the inner world of psychoanalytic training.

Analytic institutes hold weekly seminars for trainees. The first step in the curriculum is to assign candidates to read Freud cover to cover. Only when they have understood the thoughts of the master can they can move on to other theorists, or examine contemporary ideas. The didactic aspect of the program resembles Talmudic study: commentaries on a sacred text, and then commentaries on commentaries. This 'hermeneutic' tradition has little resemblance to science, where the *latest* publications are generally the most exciting.

The second part of analytic education consists of the treatment of three patients, supervised by training analysts. Each 'control case' must complete two years of analysis. (I have heard candidates complain of their misfortune when a patient gets well too soon, since when cases fail to stay for the requisite minimum period, the therapist receives no academic credit.)

The third part of the program, considered by Freud and his disciples to be crucial, is the training analysis. The process of being analysed oneself is purported to have two benefits. First, the analyst is expected to become free of neuroses that could interfere with the treatment of patients. Second, experiencing the treatment oneself is supposed to provide insight into unconscious processes, making the candidate a better therapist. (Neither of these assumptions has ever been empirically tested.)

This traditional structure of analytic training has been criticized, even from within the discipline. Otto Kernberg has colourfully described 'thirty ways' in which training at institutes can produce conservatism and crush originality.[3] Trainees are expected to swallow ideas whole, and the system is designed to subvert dissent. The early analysts were original thinkers, and most of them (not to speak of Freud himself) never went through analytic training or a personal analysis.

Even more troubling is the custom of asking a candidate's analyst to report to a training committee. Even where training analysts are officially 'non-reporting,' opinions can hardly be kept secret. This raises the question of whether the candidate can expect confidentiality and thus be fully honest in what they say on the couch. I have known colleagues emerging from their training with the feeling that they have not actually received treatment. Some go on to be analysed again. Multiple experiences with treatment are the rule, not the exception, in the lives of therapists.[4] A famous wisecrack among candidates is that they have 'one analysis for the institute, and one for me.'

The crucial problem with institutes is a lack of accountability. This problem goes beyond psychoanalysis itself. Anyone can rent a few rooms, print a letterhead, and announce the birth of a new 'institute.' Some of the strangest and least scientific methods of therapy have tried to validate themselves in this way. To choose an example from the fringe, the psychologist Arthur Janov, claiming he was bringing therapy back to Freud's original principles, created an Institute for Primal Therapy.[5] Did this make the encouragement of screaming one's rage at one's parents a valid way of treating patients?

Since institutes are more interested in teaching than in research, they function more like trade schools than like academic departments. The last chapter described one attempt to address the problem, by establishing institutes in universities. The centre at Columbia is self-financing, in that the psychiatry department only has to provide space and infrastructure. Yet psychoanalytic centres within universities are not held accountable in the same way as researchers. Inside or outside academia, when analytic institutes fail to produce data and publications, no consequences ensue. In this way, separate institutions lead to conservatism and stagnation.

As psychoanalysis has declined, so have the number of applications to institutes. (In Chicago there was no class at all in 1999–2000 owing to a dearth of applicants).[6] As we will see later in the book, psychoanalytic candidates today might not have any medical or scientific background. This pathway can only lead to further isolation.

A Personal Odyssey

My own relationship to psychoanalysis was common among young psychiatrists in the 1960s and 1970s. Although I never became an analyst, I was definitely a 'fellow traveller.' Medical school had not provided me with a rigorous scientific training. As much as anyone else, my ideas were shaped by the world around me.

As an adolescent, I had read Freud, and was intensely fascinated with his writings. (In this respect, I resembled my teacher, Heinz Lehmann.) While Freud's insistent emphasis on sexuality as the key to human nature always struck me as wrong-headed, his concept that human behaviour was guided by hidden unconscious motives was very appealing. It turned human behaviour into a mystery that needed to be solved. Then, as an undergradaute student, meeting psychotic patients at a psychiatric hospital motivated me to spend my life exploring the enigma of mental illness.

I went to medical school with psychiatry in mind. When I entered psychiatric training in 1968, I had wanted to become a psychotherapist who would treat severely ill patients. I also hoped to become an educator who would bring together the two psychiatries. Such goals were unexceptional by today's standards. But in the milieu of an analytically oriented teaching hospital, I was something of a rebel. I became known for asking too many questions and for challenging too many received wisdoms. Even so, at the end of my training, Henry Kravitz asked me why I was not applying to the analytic institute. When I told him that my primary ambition was to be an educator, he replied, 'But if you want to teach psychiatry, how can you speak with authority if you are not an analyst?' It didn't occur to him that I preferred inquiry to authority.

Though I failed to join the club, I wanted to *understand* analysis. I read everything I could: Freud, Freud's followers, and the neo-Freudians. Towards the end of my residency, I enrolled in a McGill program, supported by the analytic institute, designed for psychiatrists who were *not* going to be analysts. It provided personal analysis, as well as supervision on analytic therapy.

My analyst was Hans Aufreiter, a Viennese émigré who was a leader at the Montreal institute. We were well suited for each other, in that Aufreiter was also a bit of a rebel. He believed, among other things, that Freud was wrong about the primacy of sexuality, that most clinical problems derived from problems in interpersonal relationships, and that analysis would eventually become a training procedure rather than a practical option for treatment.

Although I avoided being subjected to formal indoctrination, I was generally perceived at McGill as a friend and sympathizer of the psychoanalytic movement. When I gave a talk at another hospital, a colleague asked why I judged all of psychiatry in an analytic framework. My position was clear enough for John Gunderson, on a visit to Montreal, to be convinced I was 'one of them.' Like many others, however, I have changed over the years. In chapter 7, I will illustrate the theme of this book by describing my disillusionment with psychoanalysis.

Psychoanalytic Revisionism

Psychoanalysts often complain, with some justice, that its critics target ideas that few contemporary practitioners still believe in. As Drew Westen, a research psychologist trained as an analyst, has written, 'Psychodynamic theory and therapy have evolved considerably since 1939 when Freud's bearded countenance was last sighted in earnest ... [T]herapists spend much of their time helping people with problematic interpersonal patterns, such as getting emotionally intimate or repeatedly getting intimate with the wrong kind of person.'[7]

This is a fairly accurate picture of contemporary psychoanalysis. Like Hans Aufreiter, its practitioners are interested in relationship problems, not Oedipus complexes. Yet what Westen does not acknowledge is how difficult it has been to get to this point, and how hard it can still be to escape the dead hand of orthodoxy.

Fidelity to Freud's ideas was expected as long as his students (and his students' students) were alive. Freud himself set the standard for the tolerance of dissent by expelling Carl Gustav Jung and Alfred Adler from his inner circle.[8] After Freud's death, the analytic movement rejected neo-Freudians like Karen Horney and Erich Fromm.[9] Franz Alexander was barely tolerated by American analysts after he wrote that the treatment might work, not through insight, but by providing a 'corrective emotional experience.'[10] In England, Melanie Klein, whose revision of Freudian theories traced symptoms back to events during infancy, narrowly escaped the same fate. But Klein was a political genius. Claiming that adult neurosis could be prevented by treating children, Klein gained unchallengeable power by 'analysing' the children of senior British analysts.[11]

Ironically, many of the changes in analysis that Westen describes were anticipated by the early dissenters. Neo-Freudians like Harry Stack Sullivan,[12] Karen Horney, and Erich Fromm pioneered interpersonal theory. This group, like contemporary analysts, was more interested in relationships than in unconscious conflicts. Fifty years ago they had to become dissidents, since anyone who failed to believe in the centrality of the Oedipus complex would run into severe trouble with mainstream analysts. Yet the Oedipus complex, that central pillar of analysis, has fallen. No one quite dares to mention it, and Freud's great idea has been quietly shelved.[13]

As long as psychoanalysis had hegemony, revisionists could be marginalized. Serious changes in theory occurred only when the movement fell into decline. Few analysts want to state officially that Freud was, in essential ways, wrong about the human psyche. Instead, new theories are added on, while the old ones are still treated with respect. Psychoanalysis is like a Roman pantheon, in which all gods are worshipped and none discarded.

Revising Psychoanalysis: Self Psychology and Narcissism

In the last thirty years, two serious attempts have been made to revise psychoanalysis. The first, self psychology, was a brave effort that did not quite succeed. The second, attachment theory, has greater potential for renewal.

Heinz Kohut (1913–81), a Viennese-born analyst, was the founder of 'self psychology.'[14] Kohut moved to Chicago after the Nazis took over Austria. Not at first a rebel, he moved up the psychoanalytical hierarchy, becoming a training analyst and serving as president of the American Psychoanalytic Association. An owlish man with a friendly smile, Kohut later noted with regret that he had been, at least for a time, 'Mr. Psychoanalysis.'[15]

After age fifty, Kohut moved away from classical analysis. His influential book *The Analysis of the Self* was published in 1971.[16] In spite of its difficult writing style, Kohut's book, and a sequel volume in 1977,[17] created a real stir, selling thousands of copies. One of his editors at International Universities Press told me that rewriting Kohut's Germanic sentences had been sheer torture. Even so, the final result was a challenge to read.

Heinz Kohut identified something that analysts had long noticed but lacked the vocabulary to describe. Patients today do not necessarily seek analysis for the relief of symptoms. (As chapter 5 will show, when people feel depressed or anxious, they have better alternatives.) Instead, analysands come for help about unsatisfying relationships and a sense of meaninglessness. Kohut attributed this shift to a set of phenomena for which Freud had coined the term *narcissism*.[18]

Just as Narcissus was enamoured of his own image, patients can become enamoured of their own psyche and their own needs. Eternally searching for external recognition and fulfilment of their dreams, they can never be satisfied, either by work or by relationships. Kohut attributed this shift in clinical presentation to social changes: as society has become less repressive, people suffer fewer conflicts, but are increasingly confused about their identity (which Kohut called 'the Self').

Kohut believed that classical analysis doesn't work for this kind of problem. He offered a sop to the Freudians by claiming that some people still suffer from an Oedipus complex, but that others (who turn out to be most of the patients coming for analysis) had a condition called *narcissistic personality disorder*. Kohut's ideas had sufficient impact to get this new diagnosis accepted into the third edition of the American Psychiatric Association's Diagnostic and Statistical Manual (DSM-III) in 1980.[19] The definition there describes 'a pervasive pattern of grandiosity (in fantasy or behavior), need for admiration, and lack of empathy.' It goes on to describe a pattern of long-term problems in intimate relationships, associated with arrogance, a sense of entitlement, exploitativeness, and a lack of empathy.

Kohut, like most analysts, saw adult problems as the result of childhood experiences. He believed that narcissism develops when a child is not properly understood, and/or when a child is traumatically disappointed in a parent. If children are insufficiently 'mirrored' (i.e., understood and approved of), they react by becoming aloof, self-focused, and grandiose. Logically, treatment needs to correct these deficits, and in Kohut's view, narcissists were mainly in need of empathy. Still, the patient has to receive *accurate* empathy. Kohut described this process as empathy falling drop by drop, eventually filling the container of a patient's 'Self.' Kohut's approach strongly resembled the ideas of the Chicago psychologist Carl Rogers,[20] who also emphasized the crucial role of empathy in healing, as well as Franz Alexander's concept of a 'corrective emotional experience.'[21]

Kohut's evolution had brought him far from Freud. Some analysts completely rejected this revisionism, an attitude that hurt him deeply. A recent biography describes Kohut as a charismatic but difficult man who often raged against his enemies.[22] Yet for many, self psychology was the new psychoanalysis that everyone had been waiting for. During the 1970s, several of my colleagues used to fly to Chicago every two weeks to obtain advanced supervision from him. In late middle age, Heinz Kohut had become 'hot.'

Self psychology claimed to explain why analysis did not always work. When faced with poor results, psychoanalysts have been reluctant to change their methods. Usually, they prefer to believe that the analyst only needs to understand the patient more deeply, after which treatment will progress. In a similar vein, Kohut published a widely quoted article describing two analyses of the same 'patient' (this was later revealed to be a covert autobiography).[23] In the first, he had followed Freud in focusing on 'Oedipal' issues; in the second, five years later, he conducted a purportedly more successful therapy by focusing on narcissistic problems.

Narcissism became a major focus for psychoanalysis in the 1970s, the same period the social critic Tom Wolfe described as 'the me decade.'[24] Psychoanalysts used the concept of narcissism to describe an unusually difficult group of patients who did not respond to standard therapy, and the idea also had a certain appeal for intellectuals.

Self psychology declined after the death of Kohut. Even the colleagues who visited Chicago when Kohut was alive gradually lost interest. This is a fairly typical sequence of events in the history of psychotherapy. Often, treatment have been based on the charisma of a single person, rather than on a method that can be readily taught to others. Such therapies do not survive. (In contrast, cognitive-behavioural therapy is a method that can be guided by a manual, and does not depend on personal contact with its founder, Aaron Beck, and so its methods have retained their popularity.) Moreover, self psychology did not generate any research. Its ideas had more impact on analytic institutes than on universities. Concepts such as 'self' or identity may be meaningful in therapy, but are almost impossible to measure.

Ultimately, Kohut may not have understood the origins of narcissism. If children are really that sensitive to being misunderstood by their parents, we should all be narcissistic. The opposite view – that children can be 'spoiled' by a lack of rules and limits – is just as likely. At the same time, self-regard and self-promotion are rewarded by contemporary society, which the American historian Christopher Lasch has described as also being 'narcissistic.'[25] The modern world, which values individualism above all, fails to provide people with a communal identity, and expects everyone to find his or her own path.[26]

Finally, Kohut failed to consider that psychoanalysis might be 'part of the problem, not part of the solution' to narcissism. Therapy may actually attract narcissists because it makes the psyche the centre of the universe. What could be more gratifying than to have one's analyst hang on one's every word for fifty minutes, three times a week?

I had mixed feelings about the self psychology movement, and viewed my colleagues commuting to Chicago with bemusement. If analysis was supposed to help people overcome their need for idealization, why fly a thousand miles in search of a guru? Kohut's method certainly did not shorten the excessive length of psychoanalysis. Empathy may have been falling, drop by drop, into the barrel of the patient's 'Self.' But the process still took seven years or more.

Still, Kohut was probably on to something. Without saying outright that Freud was wrong, he described patients for whom another theory was required, and took the position that understanding people empathically has more healing potential than a classical interpretative stance. Kohut could have stated more clearly that human suffering is less about sex and more about thwarted love and ambition. This message would not have been very different from what religious teachers have been proclaiming for millennia.

Otto Kernberg is the other great psychoanalytic theorist of narcissism.[27] Another Viennese émigré who barely escaped the Holocaust, he once told me that his father, a First World War veteran, thought himself safe, but Kernberg's mother saw extermination coming. The entire family moved to Chile in 1939, and Kernberg was educated there, after which he moved to Topeka, Kansas, and then to New York.

Kernberg is someone people like to talk about. A diminutive but powerful man, the residents at Menninger used to call him 'Mighty Mouse.' Kernberg is highly cultured and opinionated. A powerful speaker, he communicates great certainty about his ideas. At the same time, he loves controversy, and actually thrives on being contradicted or criticized.

Kernberg's ideas are fairly difficult to follow, in person or in print. (Sometimes one wonders whether ideas are considered deep when they are merely obscure.) At a meeting of the European Association for the Study of Personality Disorders in Milan some years ago, Kernberg was asked to debate with the Seattle psychologist Marsha Linehan, a cognitive behavioural therapist whose work on the treatment of borderline personality disorder will be discussed later in the book. This debate might be described as having taken place in two incompatible languages. And since no one quite understood what Kernberg had to say, it was hard to tell who won.

At the same time, there is a great deal of wisdom in Otto Kernberg's ideas. In contrast to other analysts, he believes that excessive narcissism derives from constitutional factors. (Behavioural genetic research on twins, showing that narcissistic traits are inherited, has proved him right.)[28] Kernberg is very different from Kohut, and they might even be called prophets of light and darkness. Kernberg does not believe that empathy alone can heal narcissistic wounds. On the contrary, he advocates consistent confrontations in therapy about selfish behaviour. Narcissistic people won't necessarily change when they feel understood. (If anything, they are likely to go on doing the same things but tell their friends what a wonderful analyst they have.)

As Jerome Frank showed, patients in therapy may not benefit any more from one theory than another.[29] Still, Otto Kernberg at least had the honesty to say that human beings are not 'basically good' inside. One wag, commenting on Kernberg's concept that there are some individuals who suffer from 'malignant narcissism,' remarked: 'It's good to see that psychiatry has finally found a way of describing a son of a bitch.'[30]

Revising Psychoanalysis: Attachment Theory

John Bowlby (1907–90) was another analyst who broke with Freud to develop an entirely different way of understanding human nature. While Bowlby also believed that childhood was crucial in human development, his emphasis was on the quality of attachment between child and mother.

Bowlby worked in London at the Tavistock Clinic, an institution associated with Freud's daughter Anna, and located close to the University of London campus in Bloomsbury. A gentle, kindly, and distinguished man with a shock of white hair, Bowlby was impressive as a lecturer. Once, when someone asked him how he could be positive about adults who had suffered terrible losses in childhood. Bowlby replied, with the certainty of a true therapist, 'I am *always* optimistic about my patients.'

Like Kohut, Bowlby began as an orthodox analyst but gradually changed his mind. After the Second World War, he had been asked by the World Health Organization to write a report on maternal deprivation[31] – an important issue at a time when so many children had been separated from their families or orphaned. Bowlby came to believe that disruption of secure bonds with parents was a crucial factor interferring with psychological development.

Analysts, who are not full trained until their mid-thirties, can be well into middle age before they start to have truly original ideas. At the age of fifty-two, Bowlby published his magnum opus, *Attachment*, the first volume of a trilogy, followed by *Separation* and *Loss*.[32] These three books were an ambitious attempt to link psychoanalysis with ethology and general systems theory. In contrast to Kohut and Kernberg, Bowlby thought like a scientist. Instead of making assertions based on theory or clinical experience, he supported his ideas with empirical research. For this reason alone, he was bound to be rejected by psychoanalysts.

Bowlby argued that attachment was a biological system that evolved for survival in a species in which infants are unusually dependent on their mothers. If the system does not work properly, as when mothers are rejecting or unresponsive, children will develop abnormal patterns of attachment that continue into their adult lives. Therapy involves identifying these patterns, and finding ways to correct them. 'Modern' versions of psychoanalysis often reflect his ideas.

Yet like Kohut, Bowlby had to suffer rejection by fellow analysts. He found some of his oldest colleagues shunning him. Anna Freud (1895–1983), the most powerful analyst in England, never forgave him for contradicting her father. The followers of Melanie Klein could not comprehend his interdisciplinary ideas that moved outside the traditional boundaries of psychoanalysis. Bowlby was saddened by these attitudes, but expected that future generations would see things differently.

Bowlby obtained his strongest support from psychology. A Canadian professor, Mary Ainsworth (1913–99), developed an instrument to measure abnormal attachment.[33] Under a standard condition that she termed the 'strange situation,' children were exposed to separation from the mother, then contact with a stranger, followed by reunion with the mother, while their reactions were systematically observed and classified. Unlike other analytic ideas, attachment theory led to testable scientific hypotheses and an enormous quantity of research.[31]

The psychoanalytic world did not incorporate Bowlby's ideas until much later. It only came around when its position in psychiatry and psychology was threatened. Retreating to a narrowing perimeter, analysts began to invoke attachment theory, and the research it engendered, as proof for Freud's most cherished idea: that childhood experiences shape adult behaviour and cause mental illness. In chapter 7, I will examine the quality of evidence in support of this principle.

Analytic Gurus

John Bowlby cared deeply about making psychoanalysis into a science. The analytic movement had never developed a serious research agenda, nor had it been very responsive to empirical findings. Instead, psychoanalysis generated gurus, charismatic therapists who were attractive to the clinical community but whose ideas were not based on scientific data.

Working with patients in psychotherapy is a messy and often chaotic business. The popularity of gurus shows that therapists with strong beliefs and absolute answers have a seductive appeal for confused clinicians, not to speak of patients. Some years ago, I was treating a man who taught cinema studies at a local college, and who was enraptured with the ideas of the French psychoanalyst Jacques Lacan (1900–75).[35] When I mentioned that I was not a follower of Lacan, he asked me, 'Then which one *do* you follow?' His assumption was that every therapist had to have his or her own guru.

I would most certainly not have chosen Lacan if I had needed one. Lacan was a maverick who formed his own institute in Paris after breaking with the orthodox organization. Noted for his imperious and arbitrary ways, Lacan was legendary for antics and rule-breaking.[36] He would often end sessions after five minutes if he did not think the patient was talking productively. Lacan was even known to conduct analytic sessions in taxis. And he was not above sleeping with attractive female patients. His students forgave him all these eccentricities, and Lacan always found ways to rationalize them. Like other gurus, status allowed him to get away with almost anything.

Given the obscurity of his thoughts, Lacan was surprisingly popular. Like Kohut, Lacan had a theory that the 'self' originates early in childhood, well before one can remember anything. In this respect he was a typical analyst. But since psychoanalysis came later to France than to other countries, it took on a special character there. French analysis is abstract, opaque, and in love with its own language. Some Americans disillusioned with classical Freudian approaches and searching for a new path found this sort of thing appealing. But French cuisine uses most of the same ingredients as down-home cooking.

The New York psychiatrist Robert Langs (1928–), although not well known outside of the therapy world, became, at least for a time, another analytic guru. During the 1970s, Langs was widely read and discussed, and much in demand as a speaker. A charismatic man, over six feet tall, Langs can easily get an audience in the palm of his hand. He benefited from a close relationship with Jason Aronson, head of a prominent psychoanalytic publishing house, who published his first book in 1973 (a volume that is still in print).[37]

Langs had some of the same appeal as a religious fundamentalist. As one historian of religion, Karen Armstrong, has observed, when religions such as Judaism, Christianity, or Islam have felt threatened, they have often responded by calling for a return to an imagined purity associated with the original roots of faith.[38] Something similar occurred in psychoanalysis. Bowlby and Kohut played the role of the liberal clergy, ready to reinterpret sacred texts in a modern context. Lacan was a 'born-again' psychoanalyst who claimed to be returning to Freud (although the founder of analysis would have been horrified by his clinical tactics).

Robert Langs certainly believed that analysis had fallen away from the purity of Freud's methods. In his view, therapy only fails when it is not analytic *enough*. But Langs heard 'free associations' in a special way. Over and over, he would interpret comments from patients as indirect communications to therapists about faulty technique. A tale of a frustrating visit to a car repair shop, or to another physician, was an indirect criticism of therapy. In his view, patients could not begin talking about their problems as long as they were stuck with what was wrong with the therapist. For Langs, the only true path was the classical one: to remain silent for forty minutes, and then present a synthesis of the material outlining the unconscious conflicts driving the patient's problems. Although this is supposed to be the 'classical' method, we know from descriptions of Freud by his patients that he never practised that way (unless he disliked a patient). The founder of psychoanalysis was chatty, self-revealing, and not infrequently gave direct advice when the patient got up from the couch.[39]

However much I disagreed with him, I had to admit that Langs was a canny and sensitive therapist who could sometimes be remarkably on target. When my hospital invited Langs to Montreal, we gave him a challenge, asking him to comment on a videotape of a supervision of a resident by an analytic teacher. Langs had plenty of criticism: for the resident, the supervisor, and the way the treatment was conducted. He predicted flat out that the patient would quit therapy. My role was to open a large envelope containing the chart, and read out the most recent notes. (A colleague noted that the scene resembled Academy Awards night.) I then had the pleasure of informing Langs that the patient had indeed ended the therapy, right on cue.

Langs, who was on the right politically, believed that guilt about making money was neurotic, and was convinced that patients should pay for therapy. He saw insurance as corrupting and refused to have anything to do with it. Calling his rules of therapy 'the frame,' Langs claimed that any deviation, particularly any that might interfere with confidentiality and autonomy, was disastrous. I told him that psychiatrists in Canada are paid by the government for conducting treatment (except, of course, for analysts, who opt out of the system and collect direct fees). He could only conclude that real treatment was impossible north of the border.

Although Langs criticized other people's therapy, he avoided talking about his own cases, using the justification of confidentiality. But since he never documented his results, many of his students eventually became disillusioned with his refusal to provide any support or feedback, an approach they found often caused their patients to flee. Like other therapy gurus, Langs gradually disappeared from view.

Rebels, Spin-offs, and Scandals

Therapists searching for a model that explains what they do face a bewildering array of options. By the 1970s, one could count over a hundred forms of therapy that claimed to be unique,[40] and today there are even more. Actually, psychoanalysis gave birth to many of these variants. One might begin with the rebels who broke with Freud. Jung called his method 'analytical psychology.'[41] Adler called his system 'individual psychology.'[42] These approaches, as well as those developed by the 'neo-Freudians,' were recognizable variants of psychoanalysis.

Some ex-analysts moved even further away from Freud. Fritz Perls developed 'Gestalt therapy,' a method that was designed to focus on current problems in interpersonal relationships.[43] Perls was a typical therapy guru who took full advantage of his position. A favourite of the trendy Esalen Institute in California, Perls grew a long beard, wore fashionable clothing, and was rumoured to have slept with a good many female patients. Perls's ideas also influenced a 1970s craze called 'Encounter Groups.'[44] In those days, it was not unusual to go to someone's house and find a Fritz Perls poster on the walls, quoting the guru about the value of brief and uncommitted relationships.

Even today, Arthur Janov's 'Primal Scream Therapy,'[44] a sensational therapy from the 1970s, retains some market share. Almost a parody of psychoanalysis, this approach blamed parents for just about everything. Patients were expected to relive their infancy and were encouraged to scream at their absent parents for not loving them enough.

While the methods of Perls and Janov bear little obvious resemblance to reclining on a couch and free-associating, they owe a real debt to Freud. All the therapies derived from analysis depend entirely on talking – alone or in groups. All assume that adult problems are rooted in childhood experiences, even if some have been 'repressed.' All assume that self-understanding automatically makes people more effective in human relationships. Yet however fervently they are held, these beliefs are not supported by research data.

In the last twenty years, the sequence of rebellion and creation of new therapies has continued to repeat itself. Feminists who have been critical of Freud have developed their own unique approach to therapy. Judith Herman is a Boston psychiatrist whose radical feminism led her to believe that a large proportion of neurotic suffering in women was the result of childhood abuse, and that the abuse is *usually* forgotten by patients.[46] These ideas may have made Herman controversial, but they are really just another version of psychoanalysis, albeit a revival of methods used (and later discarded) by Freud early in his career. Unfortunately, the concept of 'massive repression' runs entirely contrary to what is known about the psychology of memory.[47]

Herman's ideas sparked a popular movement. Ellen Bass and Laura Davis, humanist teachers turned therapists, published *The Courage to Heal,* a book that sold a million copies.[48] This bible of 'recovered memory' tells troubled women that failure to remember child abuse is proof that it must have happened. The recovered-memory movement created an international scandal in the United States and Canada, engendering the prosecution of daycare workers and lawsuits against therapists from accused parents, and bringing shame on the profession of psychotherapy. The creation of factitious 'multiple personalities,' using hypnosis and other forms of suggestion, is a gruesome example of the harm of which psychotherapy is capable.[49]

Fortunately, the recovered-memory scandal largely bypassed my own university. But at the prestigious department of psychiatry of the University of Chicago, an enormous settlement had to paid out by Rush Presbyterian Hospital for the practices of a psychiatrist who had been manufacturing new personalities while collecting enormous fees.[50]

Some years ago, I was invited to speak at a Canadian university about my research on the relationship between child abuse and personality disorders. My presentation took some pains to distinguish between true and false memories of child abuse. But I did not know much about the local community of therapists. Then I mentioned that memories of 'satanic ritual abuse' were a sure sign of false memories, since no one could ever corroborate stories in which babies were sacrificed to Satan and ritually eaten. There was an audible hiss from the audience, which I later discovered was filled with therapists deep into the multiple-personality cult. Later, I went home and wrote two long articles about the entire recovered-memory movement.[51] It is easier to put one's views into writing than to confront a hostile mob.

The fantastic stories of satanic abuse and widespread incest[52] (not to speak of alien abduction and memories from past lives) spun by psychotherapists in the 1990s may seem far from the mainstream. To be fair, most analysts were as opposed to these developments as I was. (Otto Kernberg has consistently echoed my criticism.) Yet as Frederick Crews has pointed out, the whole episode reflected inherent epistemological problems dating from the time of Freud.[53] One cannot accurately reconstruct events of childhood from the reports of adult patients. Nor does the 'recovery' of memories under hypnosis produce any kind of greater truth; if anything, hypnotic techniques are more likely to produce fabrications.[54]

Some psychoanalysts left the movement to support the idea that patients suffer more from real trauma than from trauma. One of these was a Canadian, Jeffrey Masson. His career path was unique: after obtaining a PhD in Sanskrit studies, he trained in analysis, serving under Kurt Eissler as director of the Freud Archives in New York. Masson broke with analysis when he began to attack Freud and his followers for suppressing the facts on child abuse.[55] This episode was publicized in an article (later a book) by Janet Malcolm in the *New Yorker* in 1980.[56] (Masson then entered a lawsuit against Malcolm for misquoting him, an action that eventually reached the U.S. Supreme Court.)[57] Masson eventually became so focused on the issue of child abuse that he wrote a book attacking *all* forms of therapy.[58] Why bother talking about fantasies when all the real problems derive from facts?

Alice Miller, a German analyst, held similar views. The idea that minor difficulties in childhood can cause serious problems in adulthood is characteristic of psychoanalysis, but Miller has made it into a religion. In a widely read book, *Prisoners of Childhood*, Miller, like Kohut, argued that parental unresponsiveness causes narcissistic difficulties later in life.[59] Unlike Kohut, however, Miller gave up practising analysis, and went on a world-wide crusade to alert everyone to the 'real' problem. Reviewing a recent book by Miller in the *New York Times*, Daphne Merkin remarked, 'Miller could be said to the missing link between Freud and Oprah, bringing news of the inner life, and especially the subtle hazards of emotional development, out of the cloistered offices of therapists and into a wider, user-friendly context.'[60]

Psychoanalysis Demystified

As a method of treatment, psychoanalysis has always had an aura of mystery that contributed to its mystique. But what really went on in an analyst's office? Patients did not always want to talk about it, and analysts were bound by secrecy. Only in later years did the method become open to the scrutiny of fellow clinicians. When Habib Davanloo, a Canadian analyst interested in brief therapy, showed colleagues videotapes of his work, the *New York Times* compared his openness to that of surgeons who operate in front of students and assistants.[61]

In chapter 2 I mentioned an incident in which a patient committed suicide after being interviewed by a visiting analyst who failed to reassure him about his treatment. Being distant and unsupportive is actually a caricature of psychoanalytic technique. The best analysts have no problem being warm and supportive with their patients. Unfortunately, neutrality can sometimes be confused with coldness, and this has led to many errors in practice. In his textbook of psychoanalysis, Ralph Greenson (a Beverly Hills analyst who once treated Marilyn Monroe) told a story about one of his students who insisted on being 'neutral' with a woman whose baby was deathly ill.[62] The patient quit the analysis, saying that the therapist must have more problems than she did. Greenson told the student the patient had been perfectly right.

The more experienced they are, the more analysts drop the rigidity and distance they have been trained to display, and act like good therapists. The problem is that for a long time, they did not write about what they really did. Heinz Kohut was something of an exception. Writing about his treatment of a patient who described driving dangerously, Kohut recalled telling him, 'Now I am going to give you the deepest interpretation of the analysis: you are an idiot!'[63]

Psychoanalysis on the Defensive

Once the main subject of analytic therapy became troubled relationships, and once Freud's original ideas were quietly shelved, the boundary between psychoanalysis and other forms of treatment became blurred. As psychoanalytic treatment was demystified, its uniqueness was less evident. Why spend years on the couch if the same goal can be accomplished seeing a therapist once a week for a few months, or even by taking Prozac?

At the same time, biological researchers continue to criticize psychoanalysis as lying outside the scientific mainstream. Eric Kandel (1925–) of Columbia is a psychiatrist who has earned a Nobel Prize for research on the synapse. But Kandel has not forgotten his training as a medical specialist. In 1999, he wrote an influential and frequently discussed article in the *American Journal of Psychiatry* about the need for clinical psychiatry to get in step with neuroscience.[64] After a furious exchange of letters with readers over the next few months, Kandel followed up with a second article making the specific point that psychoanalysis and psychotherapy have failed to keep up with advances in brain research.[65]

To redefine itself in this climate, analysis has searched for a new theory. For some, Bowlby's attachment model was the answer. Peter Fonagy (1949–), Freud Memorial Professor at University College, London, is a psychologist, psychoanalyst, and researcher who regularly visits the Menninger Clinic. Fonagy might be described as, to paraphrase W.S. Gilbert, 'the very model of a modern psychoanalyst.' Like his analytic colleagues, Fonagy still sees psychopathology as the result of childhood experience.[66] The difference is that he attempts to support his ideas with empirical data. Fonagy is a serious academic who takes science seriously. (I recently heard him lecture on the implications of behaviour genetics, which, as we will see later in this book, greatly undermines the classical belief that personality is formed in childhood.)

The American analyst Glen Gabbard (1948–) is currently the most prominent psychoanalyst working within the academic community. A psychiatrist who spent most of his career at the Menninger Clinic, Gabbard now works at Baylor University in Houston, the site to which the Menninger has moved. A dapper and charming man, Gabbard is a fine speaker and a writer of rhetorical skill. His mission is to maintain an important place for psychoanalysis within psychiatry. If anyone has doubts about the continued influence of analysis on clinicians, they should peruse Gabbard's book, *Psychodynamic Theory in Clinical Practice*, now in a third edition and a best-seller for American Psychiatric Press.[67]

Gabbard writes with clinical acumen, but plays by the rules of medicine and science, drawing on empirical evidence to support his ideas. His message, which is highly reassuring to analytically oriented therapists, is that most of their clinical impressions from practice have been confirmed by research. Gabbard argues that no contradiction exists between the Freudian unconscious and current knowledge about brain function.[68] He points out that recent research shows that psychotherapy (such as cognitive therapy for obsessions and compulsions) can actually change brain activity (as measured by such imaging techniques as MRI scans).[69]

Psychoanalysts like Fonagy and Gabbard are not content to remain isolated within institutes. They have left the fortress to champion analysis, fighting against the current academic *Zeitgeist*. They came to realize that while institutes may have protected psychoanalysis in the short run, they seriously damaged its cause in the long run. Fonagy and Gabbard attempt to find a way to square the circle and reconcile analysis with conflicting data. While their arguments are not convincing, they have agreed to play by scientific rules.

Part Two

CHALLENGE

chapter 4

Counter-Revolution

The Return to Kraepelin

Sigmund Freud is not the most influential figure in the history of psychiatry. That role should now be assigned to Emil Kraepelin (1856–1928).[1] A tough-minded academician who headed a university department in Munich, Germany, Kraepelin was born in the same year as Freud, but was in many ways his opposite. While Freud was interested in exploring childhood events and the unconscious mind, Kraepelin's focus was on precise observation of symptom patterns and the development of a valid classification of mental illness. Whereas Freud had an office practice and was most interested in neuroses, Kraepelin ran several mental hospitals and was more interested in psychoses.

Kraepelin had little respect for psychoanalysis. Towards the end of his career, he published these acerbic and sceptical comments on Freud:[2]

> Here we meet everywhere the characteristic fundamental feature of the Freudian method of investigation, the representation of arbitrary assumptions and conjectures as assumed facts, which are used without hesitation for the building up of always new castles in the air, ever towering higher, and the tendency to generalizations beyond measure from single observations. I must finally confess that with the best will I am not able to follow the trains of thought of this 'metapsychiatry,' which, like a complex, sucks up the sober method of clinical observation. As I am accustomed to walk on the sure foundation of direct experience, my Philistine conscience of natural science stumbles at every step on objections, considerations, and doubts, over which the lightly soaring power of imagination of Freud's disciples carries them without difficulty.

Kraepelin saw mental illness as no different from physical illness. He grew up during a time when medicine was making great strides in classifying pathology, and when causative agents were being discovered for specific diseases. The problem for psychiatry is that it only used a few broad categories, such as psychosis and neurosis. Kraepelin developed a new classification of disease that depended on course and outcome. His system differentiated 'dementia praecox' (later called schizophrenia) from manic depression (later called bipolar disorder).[3] This distinction became crucial for the development of modern psychiatry.

In the early years of the twentieth century, Kraepelin's influence was as dominant in America as in Europe. But as psychoanalysis became more influential, Freud was perceived as a leader, while Kraepelin was gradually forgotten. Kraepelin was often seen as a prehistoric figure who had only been taken seriously before the dawn of analysis. In his influential book *The Divided Self*,[4] the Scottish psychoanalyst Ronald Laing made a special point of criticizing Kraepelin, whom he saw as entirely lacking in humanism and empathy. Reviewing transcripts of his demonstration interviews on psychotic patients, Laing sarcastically compared Kraepelin's emphasis on symptoms and diagnosis to an entomologist's cataloguing of rare butterflies.

Yet Kraepelin never lost his influence on the continent of Europe. Before and after the Second World War, German psychiatrists, such as Kurt Schneider and Karl Jaspers,[5] focused on careful observation and classification of psychotic illness. The Kraepelinian tradition also remained alive in Britain, particularly at the Maudsley Hospital in London. There, the leading teacher after the war was the Australian psychiatrist Aubrey Lewis (who had studied with Adolf Meyer).[6] Lewis shaped a whole generation of psychiatrists who came to London to study at the Maudsley and spread themselves around the Commonwealth. Twenty years ago, many of the chairs of psychiatry in Canada were Maudsley graduates with vivid memories of studying under Lewis.

Like Kraepelin, Aubrey Lewis was a sceptic, interested only in facts. (Sometimes scepticism could become too much of a reflex, as when Lewis initially failed to recognize the breakthrough discovery of antipsychotic drugs.) Lewis had little respect for psychoanalysis. Although he himself did not publish a great deal, a textbook of psychiatry written by his colleagues at the Maudsley (Willy Mayer-Gross, Eliot Slater, and Martin Roth)[7] was an 'alternative' text when I studied psychiatry. It offered a markedly different perspective from the American, psychoanalytically inspired books we were assigned to read. Mayer-Gross, Slater, and Roth were more interested in evidence than in theory, and they dismissed psychoanalysis out of hand.

At the same time, Kraepelin was forgotten in North America; his name was rarely mentioned during my training. A revival of interest in his work was the last thing any of us would have expected. Yet only a few years later, this is exactly what happened, and the results turned psychiatry upside down. The story begins in the American heartland, at the somewhat unlikely locale of St Louis, Missouri.

The Young Turks of Washington University

Psychiatrists at Washington University in St Louis were instrumental in fomenting a counter-revolution that overthrew the power of psychoanalysis in American psychiatry.[8] From the 1950s on, the 'Wash U' group brought together a like-minded group of rebels against psychoanalysis who advocated a return to the principles enunciated by Emil Kraepelin. It then seeded departments in Iowa City and Minneapolis, and earned crucial support from psychiatrists at Columbia.

How did a relatively obscure department become the nucleus for radical change? For one thing, St Louis had never been an analytic stronghold. The medical school at Washington University had a strong tradition in the neurosciences. When the department of psychiatry and neurology was founded in 1938, the first chair was a neurologist, David Rioch. Under the second chair, Edwin Gildea (1942–63), psychiatry separated itself from neurology. Gildea had studied the biological aspects of schizophrenia at Yale, and built a department that, even if it did not exclude analysis, made it marginal.

Another important factor favouring academic medicine at Washington University was that the school had a full-time system promoting research. Even at leading universities such as Harvard and Columbia, full-time faculty could earn lucrative incomes in practice, and many only made a partial commitment to academic life. Even today, my colleagues at many American universities describe a 'three o'clock exodus,' in which clinical faculty leave the grounds of hospitals to see paying patients in downtown offices. At Wash U, however, full-timers had to return all their clinical earnings to the university. No financial incentive existed to dilute their commitment to academia.

As good as the Washington University department was, it lacked national influence. The turning point came in the 1950s with the recruitment of Eli Robins, a young psychiatrist trained at Harvard.[9] Rob-

ins, who grew up in a small town in Texas, was the son of a Russian immigrant businessman. As a medical student, Robins had developed
paralysis and was hospitalized. A psychoanalyst who consulted on the
case was sure that Eli was suffering from hysteria. But a psychiatrist working in the neurology department, Mandell Cohen, did not agree.

Robins was actually showing the first symptoms of multiple sclerosis
(MS). About fifty years later, he died of complications from this progressive neurological disease. In its early stages, MS can have a confusing
course, presenting fleeting symptoms that can easily be mistaken for hysteria, and then going into long periods of remission. Robins was able to
hide his illness when he was up for appointment as chair, and managed
to hold the job for twelve years (1963–75). Even when his disability
became obvious, he worked on heroically, no matter what state of health
he was in. Eventually, Robins was forced to resign due to lapses of memory that interfered with his job performance. In 1992 I saw him, in his
wheelchair, being honoured by the American Psychiatric Association
with its Distinguished Service Award.

In Boston, Robins had trained under his former consultant, Mandell
Cohen. A neuropsychiatrist who, like many academics of his time, had
studied under Adolf Meyer, Cohen developed an interest in anxiety and
depression. A later chair at Washington University, Robert Cloninger,
considers Cohen 'the grandfather of biological psychiatry,'[10] in that he
pioneered the medical approach to mental disorders. Cohen was hostile
to the direction psychiatry had taken at Harvard. He hated the analysts
there, who returned the favour by calling his approach 'superficial.'

Robins, although he later shared his mentor's distaste for Freud, had
once flirted with analysis. Like other bright Harvard residents, he considered entering the Boston institute. Since application for training
requires a preliminary period of personal analysis, Robins spent a year
on the couch with one of Freud's most famous Viennese disciples,
Helene Deutsch. But Robins gave up the analysis and never applied for
further training. It is also possible that Robins held a special grudge
against analysis. A close relative who developed severe depression was
treated with analytic therapy at McLean Hospital, where he died after
jumping from an upper storey.

Robins arrived at Washington University in the early 1950s on
Cohen's recommendation, joined by his sociologist wife Lee. A New
Orleans native, Lee Robins had met her husband at Harvard. She
became one of the great pioneers of psychiatric epidemiology, and her
Deviant Children Grown Up[11] is a seminal and still unrivalled study of the

childhood origins of psychopathy. Later, Lee Robins led the first major epidemiological investigation funded by NIMH, the famous Epidemiological Catchment Area Study, and co-authored a book summarizing its findings.[12] Thus, when the two Robinses came to Wash U, the department got a 'twofer.'

When Eli Robins became chair, the analysts on faculty were his most obvious opponents, and he quickly got rid of them. (This kind of blood-letting, while possible forty years ago, is thoroughly impossible today.) Alex Kaplan, a former president of the American Psychoanalytic Association, continued to teach residents, but most left quietly. In any case, an analyst could make more money in private practice than the university could have offered.

Within a few years, two other dynamic young men joined Eli and Lee. Samuel Guze (pronounced 'Goozay') was a New Yorker trained in St Louis. Guze (1925–99) had completed a residency in internal medicine, but became interested in psychiatry while working on a consultation-liaison service. Unlike Robins, Guze had never even considered becoming an analyst. He always believed that psychiatry should be part of medicine, and should follow a medical model like any other specialty.[13] Guze was not a prolific researcher, but his published work focused on making psychiatric diagnosis more precise. At Washington University, he served as head of the consultation service, and later succeeded Robins as chair (1975–89).

The third member of the triumvirate was George Winokur, a Baltimore-trained psychiatrist who arrived in St Louis in 1954. Like Robins, Winokur had originally planned to be a psychoanalyst. He was diverted from this goal after transferring to Washington University for his last year of residency. Richard Hudgens, a psychiatrist who worked with the Wash U group, describes Winokur as 'an outspoken and stimulating teacher.'[14] To Hudgens the anti-psychoanalytic reputation of the department 'owed much to the drumfire of mockery which Winokur rained down on its proponents.' He noted that Winokur was an unusually funny man, who also had a way of telling people they were wrong in a non-threatening way.

All three members of the Wash U triumvirate were Jewish. By this time, it was no longer necessary for Jewish psychiatrists to be on the same side as Freud. In addition, these men came together in the American Mid-west, where the larger culture had never espoused analysis.

Winokur's research focused on mood disorders; he pioneered the important distinction between bipolar disorder and unipolar depression.[15] Unlike the other members of the triumvirate, Winokur was a prolific writer who will be remembered in the future. The Wash U group cloned itself when Winkour left to become chair of psychiatry at the University of Iowa in 1971. Under his stewardship, over the next twenty years, glory came to Iowa. A medical school in a small town in the corn belt began to produce major leaders of American psychiatry: among the most prominent were a future editor of the American *Journal*, Nancy Andreasen,[16] and Ming Tsuang,[17] a biological researcher who later moved to the Massachusetts Mental Health Center at Harvard. Winokur, who retired from the chair in 1991 but continued to work until his death in 1997, was greatly loved; when I visited Iowa in 1999, the department was still in mourning.

At first, Robins, Guze, and Winokur were isolated, with hardly any influence outside of St Louis. The *Zeitgeist* did not favour their views, and they were often unsuccessful in obtaining grants. Rejected by the mainstream, they became more united. Robert Cloninger (one of the leading psychiatrists working today at Wash U) told me, 'They stuck together because no one else would talk to them.' The atmosphere at the Washington University Department of Psychiatry became consciously iconoclastic. Cloninger remembers a picture of Freud hung just over the urinal; he never found out if this was done by Robins, Guze, or Winokur, 'but it could have been any one of them – they were real characters.'[18] Cloninger compares their story to that of Freud's followers who formed a secret 'committee.'[19] A few determined men set out to change the world.

In the end, Washington University played a major role in American psychiatry's return to Kraepelin. Gerald Klerman, a prominent professor at Harvard and Columbia, eventually labelled this group as 'neo-Kraepelinian,'[20] given their interest in studying the natural history and outcome of mental disorders. Unlike Adolf Meyer, who had thought that all psychopathology consisted of reaction patterns to stress,[21] the Wash U group viewed diagnostic categories as real diseases.

Psychiatry's Return to Diagnosis

In the 1960s, American psychiatry reversed course, developing a renewed interest in the accurate diagnosis of mental illness. There were two reasons for the change. The first had to do with policies that affected all medical specialties. Following the thalidomide tragedy in 1962, government standards for approving drugs tightened up. The

U.S. Food and Drug Administration had the task of approving new drugs for specific medical conditions.[22] The guiding concept in the 1960s was that each category of illness should have a specific treatment, and that specific drugs would be approved for specific diagnostic categories. In psychiatry, given recent advances in psychopharmacology, many hoped that diagnosis could be made more precise. Then specific drugs for specific conditions could be tested in clinical trials.

In retrospect, these ideas were naive. As psychiatrists have painfully learned, patients often meet criteria for multiple diagnoses, creating the confusing phenomenon of 'comorbidity.'[23] In theory, this term describes the presence of multiple disorders in the same patient. Actually, comorbidity is nothing but an artefact resulting from the continued inaccuracy of psychiatric diagnosis. Patients get more than one diagnosis when they are severely ill, and multiple diagnoses only reflect this severity. Psychiatrists will not be able to make diagnoses in the same way internists do until the brain is as well understood as the liver or the kidney.

The second reason for a return to diagnosis in American psychiatry was embarrassment. A large body of research had shown that psychiatric diagnosis in the 1960s was highly subjective and seriously unreliable.[24] Patients with similar symptoms would not receive the same diagnosis from different psychiatrists. When I trained in psychiatry, this was a major problem, with each teacher trying to confirm a 'favourite' diagnosis. If everyone was using a different set of criteria, there could be no way to settle arguments as to whether a patient had schizophrenia or manic depression, or even whether a patient suffered from anxiety or depression. Discussions about diagnosis were accordingly sterile. One psychiatrist would say the patient had to have schizophrenia because of one symptom, while another would point out a different symptom. Much of the time, given the narrow range of treatment options, the answer didn't really make much difference.

A dramatic demonstration of the unreliability of diagnosis in psychiatry came from the 'New York–London Study,'[25] which documented wide divergences in diagnostic practices between American and British psychiatrists. When presented with identical videotaped interviews of patients, the Americans diagnosed most cases as schizophrenia, while the British saw the same patients as having manic depression. (Canadian psychiatrists might follow either the Americans or the British, according to which side of the Atlantic they had been trained on.)

The problem was that, in the 1960s, American psychiatrists had a very broad concept of schizophrenia. Almost anybody with psychotic symptoms, especially paranoid delusions, got the diagnosis. Even patients without psychosis might be called 'ambulatory schizophrenics.'[26] This tendency was a consequence of the break with Kraepelin and the European tradition. The British, who were still, after all, Europeans, had not forgotten such basic facts as the episodic course that distinguishes manic depression from schizophrenia. Nor were they easily misled by the presence of persecutory delusions, which, as Kraepelin had long ago noted,[27] were common in mania and severe depression.

In medicine, diagnosis is based on symptoms, but can, in principle, be confirmed by pathological findings. The grounding of diagnosis in pathology (either gross or microscopic) had been established in the nineteenth century by medical luminaries such as Rudolf Virchow, the German professor who taught William Osler. It is for this reason that teaching hospitals have always prided themselves on the percentage of their patients who are autopsied if they die on the premises.

Medical students are introduced to this relationship through the CPC (Clinical-Pathological Conference). The CPC is like an elaborate game. The physician is presented with highly detailed clinical data, drawn from a confusing case, and then asked to reach a diagnosis. The pathologist is then called on to describe autopsy findings providing a definitive and correct answer to the puzzle. (It is said that while pathologists are always right, they are always too late.) Great physicians prove their mettle by coming up with the correct diagnosis. CPCs are held at many teaching hospitals, and are published on a regular basis by the *New England Journal of Medicine*.

In psychiatry, pathology has not been very helpful in establishing diagnoses. While the brains of patients with Alzheimer's disease yield characteristic findings, brains taken from patients with schizophrenia or bipolar illness are largely indistinguishable from those of normal people with no mental disorder. Only recently, with imaging techniques, have psychiatrists begun to see functional abnormalities in the brains of psychotic patients, as well as some subtle anatomical changes.[28]

Conducting follow-up studies on thousands of patients, Kraepelin classified diseases according to long-term course,[29] a concept that became the basis of a distinction between psychotic illnesses: schizophrenia had a steady downhill course, while manic depression was intermittent. The problem was that no one knew the etiology of either disease. Nor, at that time, was there any specific treatment for either one.

In the absence of knowledge about the causes of illness, some professors of psychiatry, particularly in America, became suspicious about diagnosis. When the first diagnostic manual in America had been published for state-hospital use in 1918, Adolf Meyer was opposed to it. Even though he had been an early supporter of Kraepelin, Meyer thought that an emphasis on diagnosis made the patient's life history less important than constitutional factors (a judgment with which Kraepelin would no doubt have agreed).[30]

In 1952, the American Psychiatric Association published its first official Diagnostic and Statistical Manual (DSM).[31] This document, now known as DSM-I, was developed by members of the Group for the Advancement of Psychiatry (GAP), and was consistent both with psychoanalysis and with the ideas of Adolf Meyer. If clinical phenomena were only the surface manifestations of deeper processes, classification could not be based on symptoms alone. Moreover, if disorders could only be understood in a psychosocial context, then mental illnesses had to be, in Meyer's terminology, 'reactions.' That term was used for most categories listed in DSM-I; even schizophrenia was classified as a 'schizophrenic reaction.'

I studied DSM-I in medical school, but my teachers did not take it very seriously. It provided only the broadest guidelines for diagnosis, and lacked the specific and behaviourally based criteria that eventually characterized DSM-III and its successors. Even with the help of a manual, clinicians could rarely agree on diagnosis.

In those days, academic psychiatrists had little interest in diagnostic precision. Their position was supported by the various reports coming out of GAP. Psychoanalysts were more interested in the workings of the mind than in describing categories of illness. Karl Menninger argued that since all psychopathology lies on a continuum, diagnosis is irrelevant.[32] His view was that psychosis was not essentially different from neurosis, just a more severe version of the same problem.

The next version of the manual, DSM-II, was only a minor improvement on its predecessor. DSM-II came out in 1968, at the beginning of my psychiatric residency.[33] It had two main advantages. The first was its consistency with the International Classification of Diseases (ICD), the system developed by the World Health Organization (WHO).[34] This seemed an important issue for world psychiatry, since it would make little sense for Americans to have one diagnostic system, and everyone else to have another. (Unfortunately, the ICD suffered from the same problems with reliability as the DSM.) The second advantage of DSM-II was its decision to discard the obsolete term 'reaction' for every disorder. All the same, most psychiatrists left DSM-II unread on the shelf.

The Attack on Diagnosis

In the 1960s and early 1970s, the concept of psychiatric diagnosis came under siege. The criticism came from several ideological camps, which have sometimes been grouped together under the label 'antipsychiatry movement.'[35] Yet attacks on psychiatry came both from right wingers, who thought that people should be held responsible for their actions, and from left wingers, who blamed society for psychological symptoms.

The most prominent right-wing antipsychiatrist was Thomas Szasz (1920–), a Hungarian-born psychoanalyst. Szasz, who has written articles for the conservative magazine *National Review*, lists himself on the Internet as a 'humanist libertarian.'[36] In his view, diagnosis is inappropriate for psychiatric patients who are just ordinary people suffering from 'problems in living.' In his influential book *The Myth of Mental Illness*,[37] Szasz claimed that there was no such thing as psychosis (or any other type of mental disorder) – only people who use symptoms to avoid responsibilities in life. Szasz can be persuasive, and I was surprised to find a science professor I know respond enthusiastically to Szasz after hearing him lecture. Like so many others, my colleague had identified with Szasz's social definition of deviance.

I was a member of a group of McGill residents who, in 1969, invited Thomas Szasz to debate the future role of psychiatry. As his opponent, we picked a noted Canadian professor, Vivian Rakoff, a psychiatrist whose many talents include acting, playwriting, and radio broadcasting. It was a lively debate, and Szasz, a tiny but emotional man, became increasingly excited as he spoke, almost jumping up and down with passion. Szasz took the position that patients should be held fully responsible for their problems, and should only be offered treatment when they are free to choose it. At the post-debate dinner, I asked Szasz what he would do about patients who could not afford to pay for therapy. His response was that people who want it have the responsibility to earn the money to pay for it.

Academics of a more liberal persuasion have taken a similar position to Szasz about the unreality of psychiatric diagnosis. (The left wing and the right wing of the antipsychiatry movement shared a profound distrust of authority.) Ervin Goffman was an influential American sociologist whose most widely read book, *Asylums*, was based on observations at a large mental hospital.[38] Goffman described the hospital environment as a 'total institution' that resembled a prison or a concentration camp, creating as many symptoms as it treats. Later, David Scheff, another

American sociologist, claimed that diagnoses of schizophrenia are nothing but a way of punishing deviance.[39]

In the 1960s these arguments fell on fertile soil. The image of hospitalized patients, in the minds of many, corresponded to the classic film *King of Hearts*, set in the First World War, which presented the inmates of an asylum as eccentric flower people who refuse to share the insanity of the society surrounding them. This kind of naïveté about mental illness is still very common, although anyone who has a family member or a friend with schizophrenia or manic depression knows better.

Still another sociologist, David Rosenhan, published a widely cited article in the prestigious journal *Science*, entitled 'Being sane in insane places.'[40] Rosenhan described the results of an experiment in which a group of social scientists obtained admission to psychiatric hospitals by claiming to hear voices. They were kept for observation even though they acted completely normally once on the ward. Needless to say, the fact that one can fake mental illness does not prove its non-existence. Nor does the fact that the scientists were not immediately discharged prove anything other than the caution of the hospital psychiatrists. Nonetheless, the Rosenhan study, which was presented in a way to make psychiatry and psychiatric diagnosis look foolish, was endlessly quoted.

In the 1960s, Ronald Laing (1927–89), the Scottish psychoanalyst and cultural guru, became a prominent left-wing antipsychiatrist. Laing hated psychiatric diagnosis as dehumanizing, saw psychosis as a response to an insane society, and doubted the very existence of mental illness. Laing's influential book *The Politics of Experience* reflected the climate of the times, and was widely read by young psychiatrists.[41] Laing even promoted the value of hallucinogenic drugs, gaining this accolade from the LSD guru Timothy Leary: 'You will not find on this planet a more fascinating man than Ronald Laing.'[42] A romantic idealist who thought psychosis might be a 'good trip' for which psychiatrists should only act as guides, Laing actually created a unit for patients along these lines in London (which fortunately no longer exists.)

Much in demand as a speaker and public intellectual, Laing was idolized by the young. As the times changed, and he suffered serious personal problems (multiple divorces and alcoholism), Laing faded from public view,[43] and is now only a subject of historical interest. His ideas have little influence today on psychiatry or on the public at large.

The Vietnam War was probably one of the driving forces behind the antipsychiatry movement. Everyone was questioning authority, and it was not unusual for psychiatry to be seen as an 'agent of the establishment.' My group of McGill residents decided to organize a debate on this very issue. We invited the noted left-wing intellectual Herbert Marcuse to debate with our own professor, Heinz Lehmann. I also invited a radical young psychiatrist (whom I will call Robert), a resident known for his antiwar activism, including a well-publicized burning of his membership card at a meeting of the American Medical Association.

This event proved to be a *cause célèbre*. (It was videotaped and excerpts appeared that evening on the CBC national news.) The meeting was invaded by a group of 'Maoists' who refused to pay for their tickets, and who heckled the speakers. Marcuse accused psychiatry of being on the side of conformity and of diagnosing dissidents. Lehmann criticized revolutionaries, noting that they always promised cream 'after the revolution,' but never provided any. Robert stood up and said, 'I'll show you some,' spraying Lehmann with a can of whipped cream. When McGill's principal, the distinguished surgeon Roche Robertson, tried to stop him, Robert sprayed him too. The meeting fell into an uproar, with the Maoists screaming and threatening to march on a working-class area of the city in order to start an immediate uprising. Surprisingly, it was Lehmann who calmed the crowd, saying, 'Maybe I shouldn't have said what I did, but let's go on with the debate.' And so it did, at least for another half-hour. Marcuse defended Robert using classical sixties rhetoric: 'I don't know why you are making a fuss about whipped cream when peasants in Vietnam are being napalmed.'

Some people thought the whole incident was a put-up job planned by the organizers. But Robert had arrived in Montreal intending to disrupt the debate. I did not invite him to the post-debate dinner, but since one of the other residents had confiscated the whipped cream, we all sprayed it on our strawberries and ate it.

Twenty years later, I saw Robert's name on the program of an American Psychiatric Association meeting. Now a psychiatrist working for a large insurance company, he presented statistics on the insurability of patients with substance abuse. Like other young radicals, he had, in middle age, joined the establishment.

The Washington University Group Wins Out

Ultimtately, the excesses of the 'antipsychiatry' movement of the 1960s reflected a vacuum of knowledge about mental illness. How could we answer such attacks without being able to demonstrate biological findings to show that psychoses were no different from other forms of medical illness? Over the coming decades, this situation was to change. Developments in the neurosciences led psychiatrists, and then their patients, to believe that mental disorders were not due to psychic or social conflict, but were the result of 'chemical imbalances.'

Even before these discoveries, psychiatrists smarted from critiques of their diagnostic practices. Without diagnostic precision, their medical colleagues would always look down on them. As trained physicians, psychiatrists had to be unsatisfied with an inability to establish meaningful categories. Eventually, leading academicians in the field became interested in systematic diagnosis. Psychoanalysis, tied to antibiological and antidiagnostic models, was bound to lose influence.

In 1970, Robins and Guze published an article in the *American Journal of Psychiatry* offering a conceptual basis for accurate diagnosis.[44] They argued that any valid diagnostic entity should meet five criteria: (1) clear-cut clinical description (based on overt symptoms, not inferred mechanisms); (2) laboratory studies (similar to those used in internal medicine); (3) delimitation from other disorders (the hoped-for non-overlap of categories); (4) follow-up studies (documenting a characteristic outcome over time); and (5) family studies (which should point to a specific biological vulnerability). All these criteria were based on the assumption that major illnesses in psychiatry were no different from those in medicine, and that they had biological causes.

Robins and Guze's requirements were much in the spirit of Kraepelin. Professors on the Continent (especially Germans), had always valued exact description of clinical symptoms. Family studies and long-term follow-up for outcome had long been at the forefront of European research in psychiatry. Beginning in the 1950s, Robins, Guze, and Winokur were using this approach to study conditions as diverse as schizophrenia, manic depression, hysteria, and psychopathy.

The real breakthrough for the Wash U group came in 1972 with an article published in the *Archives of General Psychiatry*.[45] Its first author, John Feighner, was chief resident in the department; Robins, Guze, and Winokur, among others, were co-authors. Entitled 'Diagnostic criteria for use in psychiatric research,' it became one of the most frequently cited papers in the history of psychiatry. Feighner and his colleagues had turned what was originally a section of a grant by Robins and Guze into an manifesto. Using the tools that Eli and Lee Robins had developed in the fifties, they showed how classification could be made reliable. The key involved establishing observable criteria that lead algorithimically to specific diagnoses. This concept became the basis for revising the DSM system.

The DSM Revolution

The neo-Kraepelinians soon earned an important ally from Columbia University. In the mid 1970s, Robert Spitzer, an analyst who had moved into research, was in charge of the development of a new edition of DSM.[46] A specialist in 'psychometrics' (the measurement of psychological states), Spitzer became responsible for a paradigm shift. He created a task force to design a new DSM, a third of whose members had trained at Washington University. (The final form of the document was influenced by psychiatrists at Columbia close to Spitzer, with Donald Klein also playing a key role.)

The American Psychiatric Association published DSM-III in 1980.[47] Unlike its predecessors, which had languished on the shelves, this edition became a best-seller. The publication of DSM-III revolutionized psychiatry. Its use quickly spread to Canada, which in any case had always followed the American system. DSM-III eventually conquered most of the world; there are very few countries that use the WHO classification. In my own department, senior psychiatrists who had never kept up with the literature felt compelled to read and master the new manual. Seven years later a revision followed, called DSM-III-R.[48] Today, a copy of the current version, DSM-IV,[49] can be found in the office of every psychiatrist, psychologist, and social worker treating mentally ill patients. (Some even insist on the 'silver book' – the colour of DSM-IV-TR, a lightly revised 2000 version.)[50]

The central principle behind DSM-III was reliability. That is just what previous classifications had lacked. As psychologists have long known, no measure can be valid (i.e., measure what it is supposed to measure) until it is first reliable (i.e., produces consistent results). Each diagnosis in DSM-III is made by identifying specific criteria in an algorithmic sequence. Thus, psychiatrists no longer need to have arguments that stem from a focus on different symptoms. DSM solved the problem by using what has been called a 'chinese menu' approach, for instance, requiring two symptoms from category A, three from B, and one from C. To get the correct diagnosis, you just have to sit down and count. Of course, the problem with reliability is that it does not prove validity. *That* will have to wait until we learn enough about the causes of mental illness to develop an entirely new classification.

Nonetheless, it was an innovation to define disorders entirely on the basis of clinical symptoms and their course, rather than on the basis of any theory. (This is more or less what Kraepelin had in mind.) The problem with DSM-I and DSM-II is that they used incorrect theories to categorize illness. The best example was the term 'neurosis,' which had been defined in terms of unconscious conflicts. Whether or not this definition is true, such conflicts cannot be observed or measured, and psychiatrists do not even agree on what they are. This lack of clarity makes the whole concept unreliable. Spitzer concluded that there were no clear inclusion (or exclusion) criteria for such a category. In this respect, the 'atheoretical' approach of DSM-III was relatively progressive.

However, the decision of DSM-III to eliminate 'neurosis' was provocative and led to great opposition, including a threat of secession from the APA by the psychoanalytic community.[51] After all, the concept of neurosis had been central to Freud's thought. Otto Kernberg, later president of the International Psychoanalytical Association, told me at the time that he considered DSM-III nothing but a frontal attack on the analytic movement. But Spitzer solved this thorny political problem in a clever way. He placed the older terms in *parentheses*. Then, in later revisions, 'neurosis' was quietly dropped from the manual, never to reappear.

After DSM-III-R was published, some psychiatrists complained about the large number of changes in just a few years, and felt that Spitzer might have been responsible for too many manuals. The American Psychiatric Association, which wanted stability, appointed Allen Frances, a professor at Cornell, as editor of the next edition. Frances was trained as an analyst, but also had a research background, and was a much less controversial figure.

Published in 1994, DSM-IV was designed to last for fifteen years. (This turned out to be an accurate prediction: the 2000 version was essentially the same, and DSM-V is expected only at the end of the current decade.) Yet since the essential concepts introduced in 1980 remain in place, Robert Spitzer must go down in history as one of the most influential psychiatrists of the twentieth century.

Twenty years ago, DSM-III was the subject of controversy and criticism. Today the manual and its successors have become an icon. Ironically, the DSM solution to diagnostic unreliability created a new problem. We don't know if its categories are real, and reliability has trumped validity. To be fair, DSM was never meant to describe diseases in the same way as internal medicine or surgery might, but only to provide a common language for the discipline. The major psychiatric diagnoses are not 'real diseases.' Rather, depression and schizophrenia will probably turn out to be *syndromes*, like heart failure or jaundice, that can have a variety of causes. Unfortunately, many psychiatrists do not understand this. For example, DSM distinguishes between mood and anxiety disorders, while research shows that these conditions often coexist.[52] A combination of depression and anxiety may be the most common psychiatric syndrome in medical practice.[53]

Some of the problems inherent in DSM disappear once we realize that it is only a rough-and-ready map to an unexplored area. I teach my students to learn DSM thoroughly, but not to take it as gospel. A realistic view is that it is a provisional system, better than what came before it, but likely to undergo radical changes as research in psychiatry progresses.

Unfortunately, some psychiatrists are all too ready to diagnose according to the manual, and then to treat patients with a pharmacological agent that seems to correspond to a DSM category. Thus, every depressed patient gets an antidepressant, even when the clinical picture makes efficacy doubtful. (And the choice of drug often derives from the latest recommendation from the pharmaceutical industry.) This is not how DSM was intended to be used: its aim was to provide a language for psychiatry, not a guide to treatment. Unfortunately, this kind of mindless psychiatry has been seen to be a consequence of the hegemony of DSM, particularly by psychoanalysts who oppose the system. Yet were patients were any better off when, irrespective of diagnosis, they were offered the same treatment for *every* symptom?

An Invisible College

The alliance between the Washington University group, its clone in Iowa, and similarly minded Young Turks elsewhere created an 'invisible college' that came to dominate American psychiatry. There was a new climate of opinion in psychiatry, and it closely resembled the ideas of Emil Kraepelin. The neo-Kraepelinians replaced the previous invisible college, the Menninger-based GAP, which had shaped the course of American psychiatry after the Second World War.

Donald Klein and Robert Spitzer of Columbia were key players in the counter-revolution. Gerald Klerman, associated successively with Harvard, the National Institute of Mental Health, and Columbia, played an important supporting role. Klerman was a paragon intellectual who had been trained as an analyst but became a strong empiricist. He turned the essence of Freud's principles into a brief, practical, well-researched, and popular technique called 'Interpersonal Therapy.'[54] (IPT is a brief treatment that focuses on problems in current relationships.)

Klerman was also interested in biological research and, along with his wife Myrna Weissman, published many studies of mood disorders. Klerman and Weissman were among the first to show that most patients with depression benefit from a combination of antidepressants and psychotherapy.[55] Later, an important study influenced by Klerman's ideas showed that more severe forms of depression do not respond to therapy alone, and usually require antidepressant drugs.[56]

This kind of research demands the identification of a homogeneous group of patients sharing the same diagnosis. Unfortunately, at this point, this level of precision is unrealistic: at best it can only be a long-term goal. It remains to be seen whether the broad categories used in psychiatry, such as 'major depression,' are one thing or many things. Most of the diagnoses listed in the present version of DSM are a hodge-podge, and it will take decades of research to sort them out properly.

Nonetheless, DSM diagnoses are a good deal better than none at all. This is why the manual became wildly popular. Clinicians found a new order in the chaos of their practice. Within a few years after the publication of DSM-III, it was almost impossible to publish research in any journal unless the patients under study were assessed using DSM criteria. The new ethos in psychiatry also required scientific papers to have reliable and valid measures of every symptom.

In some cases, diagnosis also made a real difference for patients and their treatment. Michael Taylor and Richard Abrams were neo-Kraepelinians working in Chicago who established more precise boundaries between schizophrenia and manic depression.[57] Their research showed that symptoms once thought to be characteristic of one disease could readily occur in the other, and that the real meaning of the New York–London study was that the British had been right all along.

Decades ago, a German psychiatrist, Kurt Schneider, had listed a group of symptoms that he considered to be characteristic of schizophrenia. His authority on this subject was so great that every resident, even in the heyday of psychoanalysis, had to memorize a list of 'first-order Schneiderian symptoms.'[58] Thus, if a patient heard two voices speaking to each other and commenting about his behaviour, or believed that other people could read his mind ('thought broadcasting'), he could be assumed to be a schizophrenic. Yet Taylor and Abrams showed that typical cases of manic depression, which fully responded to lithium therapy, also showed these symptoms. Schneider, who never conducted systematic research, turned out to be wrong. When lithium began to be used widely for bipolar illness, and was shown to be highly effective, Kraepelin's original distinction between schizophrenia and manic depression was validated.

At the same time, the availability of effective drugs also had some negative side effects on diagnostic practices. If bipolar illness could be treated, then psychiatrists actually *wanted* their patients to have that diagnosis, with its better prognosis, rather than have schizophrenia, from which they were less likely to recover. The result was that many patients with schizophrenia were given an incorrect diagnosis of bipolar disorder and put on lithium or other mood stabilizers. When psychiatrists are reluctant to diagnose schizophrenia, families do not understand why their afflicted relatives remain chronically ill.

How Psychoanalysts Responded to the Counter-Revolution

Medicine and psychiatry follow a philosophy of logical positivism.[59] In that perspective, anything that can not be measured accurately may as well not exist. In medicine today, nothing can be published without valid measurement. This is why psychoanalytic papers, strong on intuition but weak on data, have almost completely disappeared from psychiatric journals. Otto Kernberg was right: the DSM revolution was indeed an attack on analysis.

Psychoanalysts had several responses to the counter-revolution. The most dyed-in-the-wool practitioners, particularly those working mainly in private offices, ignored everything. They had never thought diagnosis was important and never would. Why bother with superficialities such as classification when the truth about mental illness lay in the depths of the mind?

Analysts working in academic settings took a more conciliatory stance. DSM might be a good thing in its place, but psychiatrists had to realize its limitations. It might, for example, be useful for the psychotic patients whom analysts had now stopped treating. Everyone now knew that it made a difference if you had manic depression (in which case you needed lithium) or schizophrenia (in which case antipsychotics were the drugs of choice.) But most patients are not psychotic. For many analysts, diagnosis was only necessary to fill out the chart: the *real* work still lay in the exploration of a patient's unconscious conflicts. Yet as chapter 5 will show, analysis was now working within a shrinking perimeter, while DSM-based psychiatry was dramatically widening the scope of its influence.

Analysts working in universities were deeply shaken by the DSM revolution. Let us not forget why many psychiatrists in the 1950s had been attracted to psychoanalysis. (The list includes many who later became its

enemies, such as Eli Robins, George Winokur, and Donald Klein.)
Young people want to be where the action is, on the cutting edge. Once
it became obvious that psychoanalysis no longer had this role, defectors
were frequent. A few left angrily and noisily. Most moved on quietly,
practising and teaching in new ways without ever quite rejecting analysis. As chapter 6 will show, many of these former or not-quite-former
analysts within universities became instrumental in dethroning psychoanalysis.

chapter 5

A Shrinking Perimeter

The Rise of Psychopharmacology

The psychopharmacological revolution was one of the great events in the history of psychiatry. For the first time, psychiatrists could provide effective treatment for patients with severe mental illness. I am just old enough to have seen what mental hospitals were like prior to the change. Ypsilanti State Hospital in Michigan, where I worked as a volunteer in the 1950s, was far from being a snake pit. Yet the patients treated there did not often improve. A few recovered spontaneously after a few months. Many remained in the hospital for years on end.

Until the early 1950s, psychiatrists had few useful options.[1] Drugs, such as barbiturates, could be used to calm down patients in psychotic agitation. Insulin coma might be prescribed, but was not consistently effective. While electroconvulsive therapy was dramatically effective for patients with severe depression, it had less predictable effects in schizophrenia, usually yielding only short-term improvement.

As with many breakthroughs in science, antipsychotic drugs were discovered by accident.[2] A team of French researchers looking for a better antihistamine to use in preparation for surgery stumbled on them and thought of trying them out on patients with schizophrenia. The results were so remarkable that many experienced psychiatrists refused at first to believe them. After so many false starts, a breakthrough of this magnitude was startling.

Chlorpromazine, the first effective antipsychotic, was introduced to North America by Heinz Lehmann in Montreal in the late 1950s.[3] Once psychiatrists learned how to use this agent, schizophrenic patients, instead of staying in hospital for months or years, began to go home after a few weeks. Although chlorpromazine has since been replaced by drugs with fewer side effects, the clinical results are similar. Moreover, it was found that schizophrenic patients can often avoid relapse if they continue to take medication after being discharged. Finally, antipsychotic drugs were effective in controlling acute manic episodes in patients with bipolar disorder (also known as manic-depressive illness).

The second breakthrough involved the psychopharmacological treatment of severe depression. Before the development of effective therapy, patients with mood disorders sometimes spent six to eighteen months in hospital waiting for a spontaneous recovery. This is why electroconvulsive therapy had been a real breakthrough. But ECT was overused in the 1950s,[4] which gave the procedure a bad reputation. Later ECT was viewed by antipsychiatrists as a method of behavioural control, and it was even banned for a while in the city of Berkeley, California.[5] Yet the procedure retains a solid place in psychiatry. Even today, ECT is still the fastest way to deal with melancholic (severe) depressions. In my experience, patients will ask for the treatment if they have previously benefited from it.

The tricyclic antidepressants, first developed in Switzerland, and tested by Heinz Lehmann in Canada,[6] were found to be highly effective, and psychiatrists found they only needed to prescribe ECT in the most refractory cases. In the last twenty years, tricyclics have been replaced by selective serotonin reuptake inhibitors, or SSRIs (such as Prozac), but clinical results remain much the same. It has also been shown that patients with recurrent depression are less likely to relapse if they receive maintenance drug therapy.[7]

The third breakthrough in psychopharmacology involved the treatment of bipolar disorder. Until 1970, these patients obtained little benefit from the drugs psychiatrists had at their disposal. Although antipsychotics brought them down from acute manic episodes, patients often relapsed. These drugs prevent relapse in schizophrenia, but *not* in bipolar illness.[8]

The effects of lithium on mania were first observed in 1949 by John Cade,[9] an otherwise obscure Australian psychiatrist. Yet Cade's work was forgotten for the next twenty years. After research documenting the usefulness of lithium for mania was carried out by Mogens Schou (a Danish psychiatrist with bipolar relatives),[10] the drug became commercially available in 1970. The introduction of lithium occurred during my residency, and it was one of the great miracles of modern medicine. Administration of a simple ion was effective for treating and preventing the recurrence of manic episodes. It was almost like witnessing the first use of penicillin.

In 1970, Frances, a woman in her thirties, was admitted to the ward under my care. She had already been in hospital ten or twelve times for her illness. Frances was restless, excited, and delusional. Chlorpromazine was the standard antipsychotic drug at the time, but even in large doses it did little but take the edge off her mania. I convinced my supervisor to try lithium. It had been written about in the journals, but was not readily available, and no one had any experience with it. (The drug companies may not have promoted lithium because it is too easy to make.) The hospital pharmacy did not even have lithium in stock, and we had to send a nurse to the other end of the city to purchase a supply.

Ten days later, Frances was coherent and talked in a normal way, expressing shame and sorrow about her previous state. To be certain that the lithium was the effective ingedient, I discontinued chlorpromazine (at the enormous dose of three grams a day), and observed no change. We discharged Frances on lithium, and she remained on it for the rest of her life, never needing to be hospitalized again. This was indeed a miracle. (However, twenty years later, I treated her son for a similar illness).

Analysts initially reacted with caution to the introduction of effective psychopharmacology for psychotic patients. Then, as described in chapter 1, Phillip May's research at UCLA settled the matter convincingly.[11] Once it became clear that drugs were effective for psychosis, and that psychotherapy was not, analysts retreated from the field. After all, Freud had never recommended psychoanalysis for psychotic illness, only for neurosis.[12] The patients in Freud's case histories suffered from anxiety, depression, hysteria, and obsessive-compulsive disorder. No doubt regretting their mistaken foray into the world of psychosis, analysts once again concentrated on neurotic patients.

Nonetheless, the grand retreat of psychoanalysis was not over. Antidepressants work as well as psychotherapy to relieve depression, and they act faster.[13] Panic attacks and other anxiety disorders can often be treated successfully with antidepressants.[14] Obsessive-compulsive disorder, the subject of a famous paper by Freud,[15] is actually highly refractory to psychoanalytic therapy, which is hardly ever prescribed today for the condition. On the other hand, as discovered in the 1970s, about half of OCD patients respond to antidepressant therapy;[16] there is growing evidence that the disorder is more organic than psychological.[17] A related condition is Tourette syndrome, which begins in childhood, and which causes patients suffering from it to have frequent tics and involuntarily shout obscenities. This clinical picture may sound Freudian, but patients with Tourette do not recover with talking therapies, yet benefit from the prescription of antipsychotic drugs.[18]

Thus, psychoanalysis could not compete with drugs, even in the management of acute neurotic symptoms. Freud's procedure began to look less like a standard therapy and more like a resource-intensive backup therapy for chronic and resistant cases – the cardiac surgery of psychiatry.

The Osheroff Case

In the early 1980s, Raphael Osheroff, a nephrologist, suffered a serious depression following a difficult divorce. He became restless and suicidal. Unable to sleep, and losing weight, he had to give up his medical practice. Osheroff was hospitalized at Chestnut Lodge in Rockville, Maryland, a hospital that specialized in analytic therapy, and spent seven months there. Yet his treatment was notably unsuccessful. By the end of his stay, Osheroff was still constantly agitated, had lost forty pounds, and still experienced severe insomnia.

Osheroff received talking therapy at Chestnut Lodge, but was prescribed no medication. This regime might have pleased Elvin Semrad, but it was totally unhelpful. In desperation, Osheroff's family finally had him transferred to another hospital in Maryland (Silver Hill). There, he received a therapeutic dose of antidepressants, and recovered from his illness within a few weeks. Osheroff moved to another city, returned to the practice of medicine, and went on to enjoy a successful career.

As a result of ineffective therapy, Osheroff had lost several months of his life to no purpose. He therefore sued Chestnut Lodge for a failure to treat him properly. The jury trial ended in a large settlement for Osheroff. Eventually, after an appeal, the case was settled out of court. Although the outcome did not set a legal precedent, the Osheroff case became a *cause célèbre* in American psychiatry.

In 1990, the *American Journal of Psychiatry* published a sharp debate about the implications of the Osheroff case.[19] The adversaries were two prominent Harvard professors of psychiatry.

The first was Gerald Klerman, a researcher on depression who had been trained as an analyst. Klerman, along with other investigators, had shown that while most depressed patients do as well with therapy as with medication, the situation is different in more severe cases. Thus, in patients with a melancholic symptom profile like Osheroff's, antidepressants are necessary.

Klerman had testified for Osheroff at the trial. His journal article about the case reviewed data showing that the treatment of severe depression with medication is firmly established. The evidence is so strong, he argued, that failure to provide standard treatment constitutes medical malpractice. In his view, Osheroff was perfectly right to sue Chestnut Lodge, and the jury was perfectly right to uphold his claim.

The other side of the argument was taken by Alan Stone, a former president of the American Psychiatric Association, best known for work at Harvard in forensic psychiatry. In his commentary, Stone argued that malpractice law allows for different standards of clinical care. The treatment given to Osheroff could have reflected the views of a 'respectable minority' of physicians. Thus, offering psychotherapy alone to a severely depressed patient need not constitute malpractice.

This defence of Osheroff's treatment was a bit surprising; Stone is a former psychoanalyst who has long since broken with the movement. He later (1999) published a bombshell article in *Harvard Magazine* (a publication for alumni) that strongly attacked analysis.[20] It stated that psychoanalysis had no part in the therapeutic armamentarium, and should be entirely abandoned by psychiatrists. In view of the absence of any evidence of its efficacy, Stone argued, it can only be considered a tool for literary analysis. Thus, one might have expected him to be fairly critical of Chestnut Lodge's management of Osheroff.

By the time I interviewed Alan Stone in 2001, I expected him to take a different view of the 1990 controversy. Stone acknowledged that Klerman had won the argument, at least as far as the American psychiatric community was concerned.[21] But he stuck to his guns about Osheroff. Stone said that after his *Harvard Magazine* article came out, Myrna Weissman (Klerman's widow) asked him to write a revised opinion about the case. However, he still thought that Osheroff's recovery could have been due to a better therapeutic relationship with his psychiatrist at Silver Hill.

The outcome of the Osheroff case was discussed in every academic department of psychiatry in North America. The general public may not have heard the story, but clinical practice changed. Practitioners who abstained from offering psychopharmacology to their psychotherapy patients would now feel vulnerable to litigation. Since then, it has been rare for any psychiatrist to treat a patient with severe depression without prescribing medication.

Interestingly, as Leon Eisenberg told me, years before the Osheroff case, a similar scenario had occurred at the same hospital.[22] The patient was a noted psychoanalyst, and the story was more whispered about than openly discussed. Like Osheroff, the analyst spent many months in therapy at the Lodge, and, like Osheroff, he did not recover, even after two full years of treatment. Finally, his wife had him discharged, transferring him to another hospital, where he received a course of six electroconvulsive therapies, and recovered rapidly.

The psychiatrists at Chestnut Lodge had treated Osheroff as they did because they did not believe that depression was his central problem. Biologically oriented psychiatrists see depression as a *disease*, much like any other that medicine treats. From that perspective, depression is seen as the result of imbalances in neurotransmitter function that can be corrected by medication. But psychoanalysts have traditionally seen depression very differently. In their view, its overt symptoms are only a reflection of underlying conflicts and personality disturbance.

Osheroff had been diagnosed at the Lodge with *narcissistic personality disorder*, the condition that Heinz Kohut and Otto Kernberg have written about. NPD is characterized by excessive grandiosity, leading to serious problems in intimate relationships.[23] Analysts have usually believed that patients with these difficulties should be prescribed an extensive and intensive course of psychotherapy.

Osheroff entered Chestnut Lodge when psychoanalytic ideas about narcissism had reached a peak of influence. In this context, one can understand why Osheroff's therapists were more impressed by his interpersonal problems (this was his second divorce) than by his weight loss and insomnia. They did not treat depression because they did not have it in their sights.

As a researcher in personality disorders, I agree that personality characteristics sometimes explain why people get depressed. But once depression begins, it takes on a life of its own. Therapy has to relieve these symptoms before 'deeper' issues can be dealt with.

Another lesson of the Osheroff case is that the therapists at Chestnut Lodge retained a stubborn adherence to their model, even when the patient failed to improve. This has long been a problem in psychoanalysis. Analysts are taught to continue treatment, sometimes for years, even in patients who are not improving. The assumption is that 'change takes time.' While that belief is sometimes true, it can be an obstacle to critical review.

Tom McGlashan, a psychiatrist and psychoanalyst and professor at Yale, who worked for many years at Chestnut Lodge, thinks that the treatment given to Osheroff was clearly wrong.[24] One can only hope that Osheroff's unnecessary suffering has led to benefits for other depressed patients.

Competing Psychotherapies

Psychoanalysis made the first systematic attempt to treat psychological symptoms with talking therapy. Today it is no longer unique. Competition from other treatment methods is an important reason for the decline of analytic therapy.

With so many kinds of psychotherapy on the market, almost anyone can call themselves a therapist, and anyone can create a new 'school.' The absence of accountability and regulation means that prospective patients have few guidelines for choosing among the established methods, and are hard put to avoid irresponsible practitioners who practise on the fringe. This is why I advise most people seeking therapy to begin by obtaining a consultation from a psychiatrist at a university teaching hospital.

Psychotherapy is an art, but its outcome is subject to scientific investigation. In the current era of evidence-based practice, all treatments are subject to research investigation of their efficacy. At this point, the form of psychotherapy with the most extensive support from data is cognitive behavioural therapy.

Aaron Beck (1920–) is one of the great pioneers of contemporary psychiatry. Almost single-handedly, Beck developed a new form of psychotherapy that built in, from the very beginning, empirical evaluation of its efficacy.[25]

Beck graduated from Yale Medical School in 1946. He began by studying neurology but shifted to psychiatry, spending two years as a fellow in Austen Riggs, a private psychoanalytically oriented hospital in the Berkshires. Beck moved to Philadelphia in 1954, where he became affiliated with the University of Pennsylvania and entered the Psychoanalytic Institute, graduating in 1958.

Beck was always interested in research. His first published study was an attempt to determine whether one could measure Freud's concept of 'aggression turned against the self' as a way of explaining depression. Beck studied the dreams of depressed patients, but his findings did not support Freud. Beck felt forced to move away from analysis to develop his own ideas.

Beck told me that the group of analysts with whom he worked at Pennsylvania were well meaning but lacked formal research training, and lacked a research ethos of doubt and self-criticism.[26] Whenever Beck's data failed to confirm theory, he would be told to 'look deeper.' In later years, Beck would use a contrary one-liner in his lectures: 'There's more on the surface than meets the eye.'

Beck based cognitive therapy on clinical observations of automatic thinking and negative self-appraisals in his depressed patients. Knowledgable in academic psychology, Beck was influenced by the work of the psychologist George Kelly (1905–67), a professor from Ohio State University who had written an influential book entitled *The Psychology of Personal Constructs.*[27]

After practising analysis for the first few years of his career, Beck began to ask patients to sit up and focus on cognitive distortions in their interpersonal relationships. Beck originally thought of his ideas only as an addendum to analysis. Eventually, he realized that 'analytic theory was untenable and untestable.'[28] There was no reliability about the meaning of clinical material from one analyst to another, and the treatment method was unproven. Although Beck eventually dropped his membership in the American Psychoanalytic Association, he served for several years on the board of the more liberal American Academy of Psychoanalysis. Ironically, the book that introduced his new model, after being rejected by twelve other publishers, was put out by the main analytical publishing house, International Universities Press, for whom it made an enormous profit.

Beck's model was promulgated through the training and research program in cognitive therapy he started in 1967. Beck states that he benefited from the fact that Pennsylvania, like Johns Hopkins, had never been dominated by psychoanalysis, and that a long line of chairs had encouraged research. As elsewhere, the analysts had dominated clinical teaching. This was true even when Beck was head of resident training, and he experienced difficulty obtaining recruits for cognitive therapy among young psychiatrists. Beck's main protégé was John Rush, who became a psychiatry professor and psychotherapy researcher in Dallas.

Like John Bowlby, Aaron Beck obtained more support from psychologists than from psychiatrists. His strongest opponents, ironically enough, were classical behaviourists, a group of psychologists who had difficulty accepting a cognitive model. Behaviour therapy had long been a favoured niche for clinical psychology. BT is based on learning theory[29] and the classic work of Pavlov and B.F. Skinner. Its clinical methods often consist of techniques to reduce anxiety while exposing clients to the situations they feared. Hans Eysenck (1916–97), a noted

English psychologist, believed that behaviour therapy was effective for almost any type of psychological symptom.[30] Eysenck, who had criticized psychotherapy for being no more effective than natural recovery,[31] spent the rest of his career promoting the unique effectiveness of behaviour therapy.

A few psychiatrists joined the behavioural camp, including one notable figure, Joseph Wolpe (1915–97),[32] a South African working in Philadelphia. By and large, however, behaviour therapy was the stock and trade of clinical-psychology students. One psychology intern, who asked me for a consultation on a young man with schizophrenia, took the behaviourist view – all you need to know is stimulus and response, and the mind can be ignored as a 'black box.' The intern's therapeutic plan was to train the patient to stop *reporting* hallucinations, since this was the only pathological behaviour he could observe. He maintained that no one could know whether patients actually heard voices, since there was no way to measure such a phenomenon.

This incident reminded me of a patient I treated early in my career. In spite of a lengthy hospital stay, a middle-aged woman from a poor area of town continued to insist on her delusion, which was that she was related to the Royal Family. I told her, 'Whether that's true or not, just don't tell anyone – they might think you're crazy.' Yet I never thought that when patients learn to keep delusional ideas to themselves they stop having them.

The narrowness of classical behavioural theory now seems as historically anachronistic as Freud's early version of psychoanalysis. Psychiatrists, whose expertise depends on their ability to assess mental functioning, never found it attractive. When psychology went on to develop a cognitive theory of the mind, however, classical behaviourism was gradually replaced by the hybrid method of cognitive behavioural therapy originated by Beck. One author has even suggested that CBT, with its emphasis on mental structures, might even be considered 'a revision of psychoanalysis.'[33]

Psychologists, particularly those with PhDs, are trained to have more respect for research than are physicians. As Beck's empirical findings made their way into psychology texts, CBT research became part of its accepted body of knowledge. Only later, as medicine and psychiatry became more evidence-based, did studies of CBT begin to appear in prestigious psychiatric journals. Residents are now being taught the method. If they don't get this training, they demand it.

Beck's view of contemporary psychoanalysis is that it has changed, taking better account of reality and not focusing exclusively on intra-psychic phenomena. Analysis still attracts psychiatrists because of its humanism, but its research base remains thin. Beck believes that in the future, there will be only one form of psychotherapy, albeit with 'bou-tique' individual variations.[34] This standard treatment will probably incorporate some of the key features of CBT.

Shortening Psychotherapy

One of the main problems with psychoanalysis has always been its inor-dinate length. Psychotherapy works for most people who undertake this form of treatment. As one review of the research literature concluded, 'Psychotherapy benefits people of all ages as reliably as school educates them, medicine cures them, or business turns a profit.'[35] But is it neces-sary to free-associate on a couch for years to get better? Do most patients need such extensive treatment, or is longer therapy required only by a few?

A variety of psychotherapies now aim to obtain therapeutic results in a much shorter time than that required by psychoanalysis. CBT usually lasts for only a few months (although as patients with more severe dis-orders are being treated, it has been taking longer). Originally designed for depression and anxiety, the brevity of CBT reflects its aims: to con-trol acute symptoms that represent a change from a normal state. Simi-larly, interpersonal therapy (IPT), developed by Gerald Klerman and Myrna Weissman,[36] is a brief and streamlined treatment. IPT, while being short and focused, is mainly concerned with the patient's close relationships. In some ways, IPT resembles modern psychoanalysis. The difference is that there is little interest in exploring childhood experi-ences; instead, the treatment concentrates on current problems and practical coping skills. Unlike psychoanalysis, IPT lasts for months rather than years. And unlike psychoanalysis, the efficacy of IPT has been grounded in empirical data.

In many ways, the practical approaches taken by CBT and IPT are not that different from what therapists end up doing in practice. When I first learned about these approaches, I found myself in the position of a char-acter in a Molière play who was stunned to discover that he had been speaking prose all his life, and didn't know it. Like many other therapists, I had learned through hard personal experience to spend most of my time working with patients on problems in their current lives. Until I read Beck and Klerman, I just didn't have a name for what I was doing.

The crucial point about briefer forms of therapy is that they can be as effective as long-term treatment. Psychotherapy research shows that the greatest symptomatic improvement takes place in the early sessions, and that longer treatments tend to bring diminishing returns.[37] Specifically, about 50 per cent of patients show clinically meaningful change after thirteen to eighteen sessions of treatment, while an additional 25 per cent meet this standard after approximately fifty sessions of once-weekly treatment. Thus, therapists can expect about half the patients they see to recover within a few months, while another quarter may require up to a year of treatment.

These research findings have important clinical implications. They show that most people do not need therapies as lengthy and expensive as psychoanalysis. On the other hand, they also show that therapy cannot be effectively conducted in five sessions – which is all that some American HMOs will cover. (Fortunately, the Canadian system, both public health care, which pays for psychiatrists, and private insurers, who pay for psychologists, are both more logical and more generous.)

Today, it is taken for granted that psychotherapy will usually be short term. This was not the case in the 1970s, when a group of psychoanalysts, dissatisfied with classical methods, developed therapies that adapted analytic principles for short-term intervention.[38] These methods (associated with Peter Sifneos and James Mann in Boston, David Malan of the Tavistock Clinic in London, and Habib Davanloo at McGill) aroused great interest in the clinical community, and each had unique characteristics.

Sifneos was closest to classical analysis: his method, which he called 'short-term anxiety-provoking psychotherapy' was designed to focus on what Sifneos believed were 'Oedipal' conflicts. Another similarity to psychoanalysis was that the treatment was elitist, in that Sifneos only recommended it for very well-functioning patients. (In the brief-therapy clinic at my hospital, I have often heard it said that if we were to apply Sifneos's criteria for eligibility, we would have no patients at all.)

James Mann, who had been president of the Boston analytic society, had original ideas about treatment. His 'time-limited' psychotherapy prescribed twelve sessions, and twelve only. This method was designed to deal with life crises by establishing parallels between the patient's problems in moving on and difficulties in separating from the therapist. For this reason, treatment had to be short, while the patient's anxiety about terminating it was often the focus. Moreover, Mann was willing to take on a very wide range of patients: I once saw him present a videotape in which he was treating a working-class man who had come to an emergency room threatening both suicide and homicide.

David Malan's brief therapy lasted longer (somewhere between six months and a year). Malan emphasized the need to establish a *focus*, that is, by identifying one psychodynamic conflict that treatment could resolve. Malan, an analyst from the object-relations school, was soft and empathic, as one could see from watching his videotapes. At the same time, he was the only one of these four innovators to conduct systematic research on the outcome of his method.

Habib Davanloo was an analyst who thought that a focused brief intervention could deal with the characterological problems that lie behind overt symptoms. To this end, his methods were highly confrontational, and watching his videotapes was a little harrowing. Davanloo and his students also founded a journal to publish clinical and research papers about short-term therapy, although they never conducted formal research.

Research shows that many forms of short-term therapy are effective. In the absence of data showing that more-extensive courses of therapy have greater effectiveness, one can conclude that treatment lasting for a few months, as opposed to therapies lasting for years, should be the standard. This is the position taken by most psychotherapy researchers today.[39]

Where does this leave psychoanalysis? Research on the length of therapy tells us that a quarter of patients do not get better, even after a year. Are these the people who should be seen on the couch? These days, as one can see at the web site of the American Psychoanalytic Association,[40] formal analysis is most likely to be recommended for patients *who have failed to recover with brief therapy.* (Some of these patients may come from the group discussed above, the 25 per cent who fail to improve after a year of weekly treatment.) Analysis may also be suggested for patients who do not improve with medication. Psychoanalysis would therefore seem to be reserved for patients with chronic symptoms. It might also be recommended for patients who require major personality change. Such guidelines reflect research findings showing that most symptoms benefit from briefer treatment, as well as the public perception that when it comes to psychotherapy, less is more. Surveys show that short-term treatment is what most patients receive when they see psychiatrists.[41]

The problem is that we don't really know whether people who don't get well in a few months would do badly in any form of therapy. We also don't know if the 25 per cent who fail to get better in a year of therapy would improve if seen for longer. And you cannot recommend psycho-analysis for personality change until and unless you prove that it can actually achieve that goal.

Almost all psychotherapy research has been conducted on brief forms of treatment, lasting for a few months. The difficulty and expense of studying long-term therapy is enormous. One would have to recruit large numbers of subjects, establish control groups, and follow both for years. Add to that the fact that research is not part of the culture of most therapists who see patients for a long time. Thus, we do not have enough evidence to come to any firm conclusions about long-term therapy.

Some modern analysts are sensitive to these issues. Glen Gabbard, John Gunderson, and Peter Fonagy have acknowledged the need to obtain evidence supporting the benefits of long-term analytic psychotherapy.[42] These authors take a positive view of the state of existing research. Yet few outside the analytic community have been convinced.

There are several problems with the literature about analysis and analytic psychotherapy. One is that most studies are 'naturalistic,' that is, they follow the progress of patients in treatment without comparing them to untreated patients or to groups receiving other forms of therapy. This approach does not correspond to the usual method of studying medical treatments, which are randomized controlled trials (to be discussed in chapter 8). The other problem is that some successful controlled trials of analytic therapy have been conducted on patients receiving other forms of treatment at the same time. For example, a study of analytic therapy with borderline personality disorder (conducted by a team that included Peter Fonagy) was carried out in a day treatment program;[43] one cannot know whether the analytic approach or the structure of day treatment was the effective ingredient.

Psychotherapy of great length can also lead to problems of its own. Like any other form of medical treatment, analysis and long-term psychotherapy have side effects. One is a nasty habit of becoming interminable. Freud was the first to write about this problem in a 1937 paper entitled 'Analysis, Terminable and Interminable.'[44]

In 1946, Franz Alexander, one of the pioneers of psychoanalysis, wrote that continuous therapy over many years can become, in its own right, a kind of drug that becomes an obstacle to recovery.[45] (In an ironic vein, the novelist Erica Jong once quipped, 'Life is the disease, and analysis is the cure.')[46] Alexander recommended making long-term therapy intermittent rather than continuous, that is, allowing patients to try things on their own for a while, and then encouraging them to come back for 'retreads.' Alexander, too far ahead of his time, was pilloried for his ideas by the analytic community.

Most patients today are not willing to invest years of their lives in psychotherapy.[47] Few still consider analysis the Rolls-Royce of therapies (leaving its competitors as Chevrolets). I have long practised short-term therapy as my 'default condition,' using more extensive (but intermittent) therapy for selected chronic problems. Over many years I practised psychiatry at a university health service, where students came and went over their university years. Each time a patient returned, we focused on a new issue, or returned to the old ones in the light of recent developments.

Is Psychoanalysis Uniquely Effective?

In its heyday, psychoanalysis was marketed as a uniquely effective and powerful therapy. While other methods were acknowledged, they were regarded as superficial and failing to produce long-term change.

However, empirical work has not been able to demonstrate any unique effectiveness for psychoanalysis – or, for that matter, for any other form of therapy. To test uniqueness, researchers conduct *comparative trials.* One of the earliest studies of this kind was conducted in the 1970s by a group led by the Canadian psychiatrist R. Bruce Sloane.[48] Patients in a psychiatric clinic with 'bread and butter' symptoms such as anxiety and depression were randomly assigned to psychoanalytic therapists or behaviour therapists. The results were precisely the same for both groups.

Lester Luborsky, a psychoanalyst at the University of Pennsylvania, and one of the deans of psychotherapy research, wrote a much-quoted paper on this subject in 1975. Published in the *Archives of General Psychiatry,* it was entitled 'Comparative studies of psychotherapy: is it true that "everyone has won and all shall have prizes"?'[49] The witty title derived from a paper by Rosenzweig, published in 1936.[50] Referring to the absence of differences in the outcome of different forms of psychotherapy, Rosenzweig, quoting Lewis Carroll's *Alice in Wonderland,* called this the 'dodo bird' verdict. Luborsky's conclusion, forty years later, was that the dodo bird verdict indeed held.

Research over the next thirty years has reinforced Luborsky's judgment. Recently, Bruce Wampold, a psychologist at the University of Wisconsin, systematically reviewed the literature and came to the very same conclusion.[51] The general outcome of therapy sometimes depends more on clients than on therapists (i.e., some people do not do well

with any therapist). However, if all therapies are equally effective, therapists must be doing something right. Yet when we compare one therapy
to another, the overall skill of the therapist in getting patients engaged
in the process is much more important than specific techniques. A
famous example was the large-scale study of depression sponsored by
the National Institute of Mental Health, which found no difference
between cognitive-behavioural therapy and interpersonal therapy.[52]

The explanation lies in the concept that therapy is a relationship, not
the application of a theory.[53] As Jerome Frank realized years ago,[54] just
coming to see a therapist raises the patient's morale. For this reason, it
has even been difficult to show that experienced therapists are more
effective than novices. A famous study by Hans Strupp, one of the deans
of psychotherapy research, was originally designed to demonstrate the
importance of technique and experience.[55] The research compared the
effectiveness of treatment from experienced therapists (many of whom
were psychoanalysts) and from sympathetic university professors. Again,
no difference was found. (My research group conducted a similar study
in Montreal, and found that medical students obtained results as good
as those of senior staff.) Again, this points to the importance of 'common factors' in therapy. And patients agree. In an earlier study, Strupp
had asked patients what they got out of therapy; most said they could
not remember what they had talked about, but it felt good to be understood.[56]

The main caveat here is that these findings can only be directly
applied to short-term therapies. It is possible (although not proven) that
longer treatments such as psychoanalysis require more specific skills
than briefer interventions. Nonetheless, this line of research shows that
much of the efficacy of psychotherapy derives from 'non-specific factors,' that is, factors that are common rather than specific to any theory.

These findings help to put in perspective the reports one hears from
people that their analysis (or some other extensive course of therapy)
saved their life. Psychotherapy is a powerful method, and it often helps
people significantly. But the data suggest that even when highly technical treatments like psychoanalysis may work, the same results might just
as readily have been obtained using other, simpler methods.

The Shrinking Perimeter of Psychoanalytic Therapy

In the heyday of analysis, psychoanalysis was seen as a definitive and
effective treatment for many mental disorders. It was even recom-

mended for normal people who only wanted a better life. One common belief was that *everyone* should be analysed. Those who were 'completely' analysed entered the Elysian Fields of mental health. Anyone who continued to have symptoms, or who suffered any serious difficulty in life, had to have been 'incompletely' analysed.

Again, this had not been Freud's view. He had originally recommended psychoanalysis only as a treatment for neurosis.[57] (As discussed in chapter 4, since DSM-III, the term 'neurosis' is no longer used in psychiatry; it was in any case a grab-bag that included a very wide range of symptoms: anxiety, phobias, obsessions and compulsions, conversions, and depression.)

Moreover, over recent decades, neuroses of all kinds have been successfully treated in other ways: with drugs, with behaviour therapy, or with both. These treatments, which are briefer and have proved effective, have become the standard approaches to neurotic symptoms. Analysis has had to search for another niche. As we have seen, practitioners had to withdraw from the treatment of psychoses. Thus, the question remained: For which conditions can analytic treatment still be recommended?

Let us examine the specific comments appearing on the web site of the American Psychoanalytic Association:

> The person best able to undergo psychoanalysis is someone who, no matter how incapacitated at the time, is basically, or potentially, a sturdy individual. This person may have already achieved important satisfactions – with friends, in marriage, in work, or through special interests and hobbies – but is nonetheless significantly impaired by long-standing symptoms: depression or anxiety, sexual incapacities, or physical symptoms without any demonstrable underlying physical cause. One person may be plagued by private rituals or compulsions or repetitive thoughts of which no one else is aware. Another may live a constricted life of isolation and loneliness, incapable of feeling close to anyone. A victim of childhood sexual abuse might suffer from an inability to trust others. Some people come to analysis because of repeated failures in work or in love, brought about not by chance but by self-destructive patterns of behavior. Others need analysis because the way they are – their character – substantially limits their choices and their pleasures. And still others seek analysis definitively to resolve psychological problems that were only temporarily or partially resolved by other approaches.[58]

This description focuses on several crucial points. First, you have to

be fairly healthy (or at least to have been healthy in the past) to be analysed. Seriously ill patients need not apply. Second, symptoms have to be
chronic rather than recent. Analysts don't really want to compete with
Prozac. Third, analysis should be considered following treatment failures with other methods.

If patients with acute problems should be referred for other forms of
treatment, then most people seeking help are unsuitable for psychoanalysis. Analysts specialize in chronic disorders, particularly those not
susceptible to pharmacotherapy. As noted in previous chapters, psychoanalysis is being marketed like cardiac surgery: a treatment requiring
enormous resources, to be used when ordinary measures fail.

Psychoanalysis and Personality Disorders

There is one group of conditions that precisely meets the bill of chronic-
ity and of failure to respond to medication. Psychiatrists call them *personality disorders*. In DSM-IV, they were described as enduring behavioural
patterns that begin early in life, that become inflexible and pervasive,
and that cause significant dysfunction in work and relationships.[59]

If we apply the DSM system to the problems described in the American Psychoanalytic Association guidelines, analysts must be spending
most of their time treating these patients. Personality disorders are the
very type of problems for which people usually seek to be analysed. They
are a last bastion within the shrinking perimeter of conditions believed
to be suitable for psychoanalytic treatment.

The German psychiatrist Kurt Schneider described personality disorders as part of a spectrum of conditions related to serious mental illness.[60] However, the literature on personality disorders became strongly
associated with psychoanalysis. Ironically, Freud had never thought
about his patients in these terms; he saw most psychological problems as
'neuroses' arising from unconscious conflicts. For Freud, people either
had a bad character (in which case they were not analysable), or a good
one, albeit spoiled by neurotic symptoms.

The first person to write about personality disorders as a unique problem was a psychoanalyst who was, at the very least, a crank. Wilhelm
Reich (1892–1957), an early follower of Freud, broke with him, first
turning to Marxism, and then moving into what we would today call a
kind of 'new age' mysticism.[61] In his younger days, however, Reich had
written a seminal book about personality disorders, which he described
as a 'character armour' that people could use to protect themselves

against neurosis.[62] (Reich's description of narcissistic personality could still be used in any contemporary textbook.)

In his later years, working in a small Maine town, Reich came to believe a number of fantastic things: that he could contact UFOs that were influencing the course of human history, and that he had discovered a cure for all human diseases. The 'cure' consisted of an 'orgone box,'[63] a wooden structure supposedly filled with psychic energy. This discovery (or, more specifically, Reich's attempt to make money by shipping his boxes across state lines) led to his prosecution by the federal government, landing Reich in prison, where he died.

Personality disorders remained the province of psychoanalysis until fairly recently. Much has been written about a condition called *borderline* personality disorder (BPD).[64] This is a chronic syndrome characterized by serious impulsivity, emotional instability, and highly unstable relationships. Unfortunately, 'borderline' is one of several confusing misnomers in psychiatry (another is schizophrenia, literally meaning 'split head'). The use of this term was based on the old psychoanalytic belief that all psychopathology is on a continuum, so that some patients lie on a border between psychosis and neurosis.

Adolf Stern, a New York analyst, was the first person to describe borderline personality, in 1938.[65] Stern was trying to explain why some patients do badly in psychoanalysis. He described a group that showed features such as 'psychic bleeding,' impulsive behaviour, and psychotic tendencies. Although Stern did not use the word borderline, his is still as good a definition as any. For the next thirty years, analysts were the only people interested in this kinds of patient. They proposed all kinds of theories about what caused borderline personality, mostly having to do with problems in early childhood. With his practical bent, Heinz Lehmann was dismissive of the whole idea, telling me, 'Don't use that diagnosis – no one knows what it means.'

The concept of personality disorders found its way into mainstream psychiatry when some psychoanalysts conducted research in the area. In the 1960s, Roy Grinker of Chicago was the first to do empirical work on borderline patients, and to follow their course over time.[66] John Gunderson of Harvard then showed how borderline personality disorder could be diagnosed reliably using structured interviews,[67] leading to the acceptance of the concept in DSM-III.

Although borderline personality disorder happens to be my own area of research, I must acknowledge a serious problem with the overall concept of personality disorder. Everyone has a personality, and everyone has problems in life. So at what point do you diagnose a disorder? Psychoanalysts have a way of considering everyone pathological, and of recommending analytic therapy for just about every problem in life. Doesn't the concept of personality disorder give them licence to go on doing this sort of thing?

Few would argue that the sickest cases, chronically suicidal patients with borderline personality disorder, do not have a mental illness. Like many other diagnoses in psychiatry, however, personality disorder blends into normality at the edges. Surveys based on DSM criteria have found that *10 per cent* of the population meets the formal criteria for a personality disorder.[68] This finding, while consistent with the current diagnostic system, does not really make sense, and we probably need to narrow down the whole concept. Otherwise, we could be agreeing with the psychoanalysts that almost everybody is pathological, and that almost everyone needs treatment.

The diagnosis of a personality disorder is most useful as a sign of future trouble. These patients often do more poorly in treatment, whether that consists of therapy or drugs.[69] Patients with personality disorders are presented at virtually every case conference, usually by befuddled juniors seeking guidance from wise seniors.

Psychiatrists cannot avoid seeing patients with personality disorders. In some surveys, they represent 25 per cent of their clientele.[70] They constitute a potential niche for psychoanalytic therapy. Several analysts have specialized in these disorders, including the former president of the International Psychoanalytic Association, Otto Kernberg of Cornell.[71]

Yet even here, in what should be its element, psychoanalysis has had to retreat. The top researchers on personality disorders, such as John Gunderson and Allen Frances, have accepted the rules of academic psychiatry, demand evidence for conclusions, and do not rely on clinical opinion. This hard-nosed approach is apparent in the published American Psychiatric Association guidelines (2001) for the treatment of borderline personality disorder,[72] edited by John Oldham, an analyst who was working at Columbia at the time of publication. Further recognition for research in this area has come from the National Institute of Mental Health, which has supported a multi-million-dollar, multi-site project to follow such patients over time.[73]

Even here, the final insult to psychoanalysis is that cognitive-behaviour therapists have been muscling into their territory. Ironically, while psychoanalysts brought personality disorders to the attention of psychiatry, their methods may not be particularly effective for these patients.

Research shows that about two-thirds of borderline patients drop out within a few months if offered long-term analytic therapy.[74]

The contemporary guru of borderline personality disorder treatment is Marsha Linehan, who is an avowed opponent of psychoanalysis. A cognitive psychologist and professor at the University of Washington, Linehan, conducted an NIMH-sponsored controlled trial of her form of CBT ('dialectical behavior therapy').[75] Although by no means a cure, a year of therapy markedly reduces wrist-slashing, overdoses, and hospital-emergency-room visits. In the last ten years, the charismatic Linehan has lectured and taught all over North America. Her method is now used and is being studied in several major universities, including Columbia, Cornell, and Toronto.

The last bastion of psychoanalysis may be falling. The long-term personality problems for which psychoanalysis is still prescribed are being taken over by cognitive-behavioural therapists, and they are starting to prove that their methods work. If this trend continues, academic psychiatry may not be exclusively dependent on analysts for teaching psychotherapy.

Psychoanalysis and Psychiatric Training

As other therapies obtained stronger data in their favour than psychoanalysis, academics took notice. CBT and interpersonal therapy (IPT) began to encroach on the special niche that analysis had long held in psychiatric education. After it has lost the competition with drug therapy, and later with cognitive therapy, the question is no longer whether psychoanalysis is at the centre of psychiatry. It is whether psychiatrists today can expect to be taught *anything* about psychoanalysis.

Psychiatry was attractive to medical students in the 1960s because it was the only way to be a therapist. In those days, that usually meant studying psychoanalysis. As psychiatry has become more focused on drug treatment, residents spend more time treating psychosis and other severe mental disorders, and less time conducting therapy. Some departments maintain only minimal programs for psychiatrists to learn how to be psychotherapists.

Yet how much do psychiatrists really need to be trained as therapists? Fewer graduates of residency programs are opening up offices to conduct this kind of practice. Young psychiatrists today tend to concentrate on hospital work. Busy with acutely and chronically ill patients, they hardly have the time or the interest to carry out extensive psychotherapy. That task is being given over to psychologists and social workers, who provide most of the services utilized by therapy clients across North America.

Chapter 1 described a debate between Heinz Lehmann and Henry Kravitz about these issues. In 1985, Lehmann expanded his views in a lecture to the Canadian Psychiatric Association (later published) enti- tled 'The future of psychiatry: progress – mutation – or self destruct?'[76] Lehmann argued that psychiatrists needed to change their role from that of expert psychotherapists to managers of acute and emergency care, and to carry out less direct treatment by becoming consultants to the mental-health community. In his vision, psychiatrists would not need to know that much about therapy, but would have a profound knowl- edge of psychiatric symptoms.

There can be no doubt that psychiatry is heading in this direction. But has the pendulum swung too far? Are psychiatrists becoming DSM robots and pill-pushers? If so, we need to take a hard look at how we are training the next generation of psychiatrists.

A few years ago, an anthropologist, Tania Luhrmann published a pro- vocative book, *Of Two Minds*, that described the inside story of contem- porary residency training in psychiatry.[77] Luhrmann, the daughter of a psychoanalyst, spent several years observing psychiatric education at American hospitals. She described two main streams in contemporary psychiatry: analysis and psychopharmacology, and saw the current trend for psychiatrists to mainly prescribe drugs (with little time to talk to patients), as a direct result of the absence of psychoanalytic teaching in training programs.

Luhrmann's book attracted a good deal of notice in the media, earn- ing prominent reviews in the *New York Times* and the *New Yorker*. Review- ing it for the *Weekly Standard Magazine*, Paul McHugh, then chair of psychiatry at Johns Hopkins, remarked:

> Luhrmann has produced ... a bleak assessment of contemporary psychiat- ric education. Casting her eye on the 'enculturation' of young psychiatrists into their profession, she argues that the recent discoveries in biomedi- cine, which the public may think are great advances, have in fact plucked the 'soul' from psychiatry, leaving it a cold business that dispenses magical pills rather than addressing patients in all their tragic particularity.[78]

While McHugh acknowledged that Luhrmann had made an impor- tant point about the deficiencies of contemporary practice, however, he criticized her overly nostalgic view of the heyday of psychoanalysis:

Luhrmann champions psychoanalytic teaching as fundamental to the training of young psychiatrists. In this, she is simply mistaken. We can no more return to the old orthodoxy than Russia can revive the Soviet Union. Luhrmann fails to appreciate that psychiatry is well free of the dominance of a conjectural theory that cheated many patients out of helpful treatment and caused a great many talented students to waste years of their lives on fruitless study.

Thus, whether psychoanalysis is being replaced by psychopharmacology is not the only question. The larger issue is whether psychiatrists should be expert in other psychotherapies that have a more scientific basis.

Forty years ago, trainees might spend at least half their time conducting long-term psychotherapy. This was considered their 'real' work, preparing them for a career in private practice. In fact, practising psychiatrists, even those working in hospitals, spent a great deal of their time conducting office psychotherapy.

Today, residents learn how to be psychiatrists in a very different way. They are exposed to a wide range of settings, in more than one hospital or clinic. These experiences prepare them for a broader and different form of practice. Their training reflects the expectation that most psychiatrists will work in institutional settings rather than in private offices. Residents usually begin by learning to manage hospitalized patients with psychoses or severe depression. In-patient psychiatry requires mastery in the use of drugs, as well as sensitive management of severely ill patients and their families. Residents then spend time in out-patient clinics, where psychotherapy is usually combined with the administration of medication. Consultation-liaison psychiatry, in which residents are asked to evaluate medical and surgical patients, is an experience that blends the two psychiatries. Even child psychiatry, once a bastion of psychoanalysis, now requires extensive skills in pharmacology.

Is there room in the curriculum for learning how to be a therapist? Current standards require residents in psychiatry to gain experience with many kinds of psychotherapy during their training.[79] This usually means they have some exposure to long-term therapy (usually confined to one or two cases), a broader experience in short-term therapy (including formal methods such as CBT and IPT, as well as less formal procedures, described as 'supportive therapy'), as well as group and family therapy. Thus, psychiatrists do not need an analytic training to become expert therapists. Yet there is a real danger that psychiatric residents are being trained to become psychopharmacological technicians rather than humanistic physicians. Almost all the academic psychiatrists I interviewed were concerned about the problem, and so am I. But the problems of the present cannot be solved by going back to the past. Psychiatry should integrate psychotherapy into training and practice, but it need not return to Freud.

chapter 6

Transition and Takeover

The Anatomy of Revolution

A remarkable fact about the decline of psychoanalysis in academic psychiatry is how many analysts were instrumental in making the revolution happen. Of course, not all psychoanalysts think the same way. In my experience, they fall into three groups. The first are those whose professional life centres around the institute and whose main ambition is to teach their craft and to become a training analyst. These constitute the most loyal troops of the movement. While many of these analysts retain part-time faculty appointments, they do not play a strong role in academia, and many work entirely outside the university.

A second group of psychiatrists entered analytic training primarily to further their careers, at a time when doing so was useful. These academics never had the same level of commitment to the movement, and many lost interest after they graduated. When the wind shifted, these psychiatrists had little problem in switching to biological models; some are barely recognizable as psychoanalysts.

A third group had been idealistically attracted to analysis as an avant-garde treatment for severely ill patients. This belief led to disillusionment when the method failed to deliver the expected results. Most continued as members of analytic societies, even if they rarely attended meetings. These psychiatrists generally have an eclectic approach to psychotherapy, and accept a biological perspective on mental illness.

The last two groups moved with the times and became academic leaders. They played a major role in changing psychiatry by allying themselves with the new generation of biological researchers. While some had set out to reform and modernize psychoanalysis, their efforts were really the beginning of the end.

In other revolutionary situations, insiders have turned into radicals. In his classic book *The Anatomy of Revolution*,[1] the historian Crane Brinton (1898–1968) observed that political revolutions tend to occur when the existing elite no longer believes in the legitimacy of the old regime. Then the change process becomes directed by people whose loyalty has shifted from the old to the new order. Recently, we have seen a dramatic example of this process in Russia. Communism collapsed when reformers such as Mikhail Gorbachev concluded that the system needed radical change. The process ended with a new government, led by former party members.

Social Psychiatry: Society as the Patient

Chapter 1 described how psychiatry has been divided into two. With the emergence of social psychiatry, it shattered into three pieces. While this movement never took the extreme position of 'antipsychiatry' (described in chapter 5), social psychiatry attracted many recruits during the 1960s, some of whom came from the analytic community.

Fred Goodwin, who has enjoyed a distinguished career in biological research, provided me with some acute observations about this story.[2] Goodwin came to the National Institute of Mental Health (NIMH) in 1964 as a young psychiatrist, and eventually rose to be director. He now hosts *The Infinite Mind*, a program on National Public Radio about psychiatry and psychology. Although Goodwin is not an analyst, his program has included sympathetic discussions of the role of psychoanalytic therapies.

Goodwin saw the switch from analysis to biological psychiatry as, paradoxically, *less* radical compared to the attractions of social commitment. Biological psychiatry, in its early days, was not much of a contender for the minds of young psychiatrists. Drug treatments were mostly empirical; psychopharmacology only became intellectually stimulating later, when drug actions were explained through neurotransmitter activity.

For Goodwin, the larger struggle of the 1960s was between medicine and social activism. Social psychiatry gained profound influence on psychiatry, challenging the medical model and its focus on individual patients. 'Community psychiatry' was an avant-garde movement that aimed to make society itself more healthy. These ideas fit in well with the spirit of the time.

Goodwin also describes how the struggle between social and traditional psychiatry played itself out within NIMH. A strong lobby aimed to keep the organization from falling under the larger umbrella of the National Institutes of Health; a formal separation was approved in 1967, which lasted until 1992. The real agenda of the separation was to protect the social mission of the Institute from mainstream medicine.

From a contemporary perspective, the hijacking of a national research centre to promote an agenda of social change seems incredible. But NIMH was not always the mecca of laboratory science it is today; inevitably, the institution reflected the *Zeitgeist*.

Since then, mainly for lack of measurable results, the more grandiose hopes of social psychiatry have been discredited. Yet in those heady days, psychiatrists were keen to change the world. This was a time when prominent leaders of psychiatry were considered to be experts about almost every aspect of human nature, and seen as pundits whose opinions were often in the media. Unfortunately, many believed the hype.

Roy Grinker was an effective critic of the excesses of community and social psychiatry.[3] Yet in the autumn of 1968, when Grinker came to speak in Montreal, he claimed that the recent riots at the Democratic Party convention in Chicago could have been prevented, 'if only they had asked us to help.' I was never clear how Grinker's psychiatric expertise could have been useful to Mayor Daley in responding to a massive antiwar protest.

Social psychiatrists believed that poverty and social disruption were the real causes of psychological symptoms. There is evidence that social disadvantage is a risk factor for some mental disorders.[4] However, the spirit of the 1960s led some psychiatrists to believe that society, not the individual, should be the 'patient.' This view contrasted with the outlook of analysts, as well as that of biological psychiatrists, who adhered to a traditional medical model in which sick people are treated for diseases.

The career of Gerald Caplan is a good example of the rise of social psychiatry. Caplan, a Harvard professor, had a background both in psychoanalysis and in child psychiatry. His 1961 book, ambitiously titled *The Prevention of Mental Disorders in Early Childhood*, promulgated the idea that psychiatrists could prevent illness by teaching mothers how to raise their infants properly.[5] Like Benjamin Spock (himself a passionate supporter of psychoanalysis),[6] Caplan saw good parenting in the early years as the key to mental health. These ideas remain alive in a field called 'infant psychiatry,'[7] in which psychiatrists work to help disadvantaged mothers raise temperamentally difficult babies.

Child psychiatry tends to produce social activists because it is frustrating work. Child psychiatrists come face to face with troubled families and troubled communities. Children, who are hard to talk to, often seem to be victims of circumstance. Most patients come from dysfunctional families and disadvantaged neighbourhoods. As a resident, I found child psychiatry more dispiriting than inspiring, and there is still a chronic shortage of physicians entering this subspecialty.[8] In my experience, many child psychiatrists do not continue treating children, but gravitate towards teaching and to therapy with adults.

Caplan was one of the founders of a model of community intervention called *crisis intervention*,[9] an approach he taught to social workers. The theory was that when patients come in a state of crisis, this is an ideal opportunity for them to change. (The concept of crisis intervention is still current in psychiatry, although today is as likely to refer to a rapid drug prescription as to a series of therapy sessions.)

But Caplan went one step further, applying his model to political conflict. In the 1970s he gave a lecture in Montreal describing his work in Jerusalem, where he was working with Israelis and Arabs to iron out their conflicts. Caplan, a charismatic speaker, probably convinced many in the audience (although twenty-five years on, the state of the Middle East conflict does not seem to confirm the effectiveness of his interventions). After the lecture, Caplan was brought up short by his discussant, the Canadian psychiatrist Zbigniew (Bish) Lipowski, who icily asked the speaker how he could possibly justify spending time on political issues when patients in hospitals were receiving inadequate care.

On the positive side, social psychiatry elicited a lot of interest in community care, as opposed to the incarceration of seriously ill patients in asylums. But the social-psychiatry movement suffered from grandiose and unachievable goals. Moreover, in dealing with issues such as the quality of parenting and social networks psychiatry moved away from its roots, and so the social-psychiatry movement became still another way to abandon the care of the mentally ill. In the end, psychiatry had to return to its proper place in medicine.

Many who had been inspired by the ideals of the social-psychiatry movement moved on to more practical goals: caring for sick people, teaching others how to do so, and expanding the frontiers of knowledge about mental illness. My own experience with social activism included a period of service in the American Peace Corps in south India. When I revisited my old site some years ago, the local people had solved many of their problems without officious foreign help. The lesson I learned also turned out to be applicable at home. Well-meaning social engineers can be irrelevant, and sometimes can even be an impediment to progress. Caring for the sick may be a greater service than trying to change the world.

Putting Psychiatry Back Together Again

The divisions between the two (or three) psychiatries were disturbing to many academic psychiatrists. Many have sought to put psychiatry back together into one discipline, and to bring it back into the medical mainstream. In the 1960s, George Engel, a professor from the University of Rochester, suggested an approach to mental illness that linked biology, psychoanalysis, and social theory into a single model.[10] Engel was a psychoanalyst with training as an internist, and was best known as an expert in consultation psychiatry. He offered a *biopsychosocial model* in which mental disorders arise from a combination of factors: biological vulnerability, psychological stressors, and social adversity.

The term 'biopsychosocial' became very popular, to the point of becoming something of a buzz word. The concept is still invoked to support broad theoretical models of mental illness, or to describe combining pharmacology, psychotherapy and rehabilitation in treatment. Engel has been endlessly quoted by other psychiatrists (including me) who want to heal the divisions within psychiatry. As a general theory of mental illness, however, the biopsychosocial model is flawed. One cannot add up brain chemistry, life experience, and the social environment. The hard questions have to do with how these factors interact. The answers will require decades of research.

To bring psychiatry back into medicine, we need research into the causes and treatment of mental disorders. But this is an expensive business. Progress is not possible without a strong government commitment. Canada has had a powerful federal granting agency (the Medical Research Council, now reorganized as the Canadian Institutes for Health Research) to provide grants for medical research. The U.S. National Institutes of Health (NIH) added another element: the building of well-funded laboratories located in Bethesda, Maryland, a suburb of Washington.

In 1946, the American Congress created a new division of the NIH, the National Institute of Mental Health.[11] Its mandate was to fund education and research into mental illness. After the Second World War, the NIH set out to recruit top people in every field. In psychiatry, this meant hiring leading psychoanalysts, such as the first director of NIMH (1949–64), Robert Felix. Felix then hired people like Robert Cohen, a close colleague of Frieda Fromm-Reichmann at Chestnut Lodge, who believed that family dysfunction was a cause of bipolar illness.[12]

As discussed in chapter 1, the idea that families can make their children psychotic was mainstream psychiatric theory in the 1950s. Lyman Wynne, a prominent figure at NIMH, was one of the main proponents of this belief, arguing that schizophrenia was the result of pathological family interactions.[13] In the context of the time, Wynne was a sophisticated researcher, and his conclusions that the families of schizophrenic patients had abnormal communication patterns were backed up by data. Fred Goodwin remembers his own excitement at the uncanny ability of Wynne's collaborator Margaret Singer to identify the relatives of schizophrenics, just by the way they talked.[14] Today, Goodwin realizes that Singer was only 'picking up the genetic spectrum.'[15]

Goodwin enjoyed a piece of luck when he came for his interviews at NIMH. Due to a secretarial mix-up, Wynne was out of town, and Goodwin was interviewed by William Bunney. An analytically trained young psychiatrist from Yale, Bunney had already 'made the switch,' becoming a leader in biological research on depression.[16] Goodwin was so inspired by this work on neurotransmitters that he forgot all about Wynne, and agreed to work with Bunney, leading to a long research career as a biological psychiatrist.

Over the coming years, the NIMH evolved into the organization it is today, the primary centre in America for research in biological psychiatry. In 1970 Julius Axelrod, an NIMH researcher, won the Nobel Prize in Physiology or Medicine for research into the chemistry of nerve transmission;[17] NIMH research funds later supported several other Nobelists.

Starting in the 1970s, the NIMH also led research in psychiatric epidemiology, conducting large-scale studies on the prevalence of mental disorders in the community.[18] The results demonstrated the scale of the problem facing psychiatry: at least one out of three Americans will have a clinically significant mental disorder in their lifetime. Finally, NIMH has been prominent in research on psychiatric treatments, as in its large-scale multi-site study of depression (whose results showed why Chestnut Lodge had mistreated Raphael Osheroff).[19]

Today, the laboratories in Bethesda, supported by generous federal funds, are a shrine for research in psychiatry. The biological revolution has changed the qualifications for a director of NIMH. No one could aspire to this position without a strong background in brain research.

After Felix, the next two directors, Stanley Yolles (1964–70) and Bertram Brown (1970–7) were researchers in drug abuse. They were followed by two analysts who made the switch to biological psychiatry: Herbert Pardes (1977–84) and Shervert Frazier (1984–6). By the end of the 1980s, the NIMH was appointing directors, such as Lewis Judd (1988–92) and Fred Goodwin (1992–4), who had spent their professional lives in research. Steven Hyman (1994–2002) conducted research on synaptic transmission, and the current director, Tom Insel, studies the links between genes and behaviour. As we will see, this is also the kind of background now required of chairs of psychiatry at major universities.

Danny Freedman and 'The Archives'

Chapter 1 described the evolution of the *American Journal of Psychiatry* from a forum for clinical opinion into a truly scientific publication. Another journal, the *Archives of General Psychiatry*, although read less often, earned even higher prestige. The influence of medical journals can be determined by an 'impact factor,' which measures how often the articles they publish are quoted elsewhere. *Lancet* and the *New England Journal of Medicine* have the highest impact factors in medicine, while *Archives* is the clear leader in psychiatry.

In 1958, Roy Grinker, the eclectic psychoanalyst from Chicago, founded a new journal, sponsored by the American Medical Association (replacing an earlier publication, the AMA *Archives of Psychiatry and Neurology*). The word 'general' in its title meant that *Archives* would address the needs of the larger psychiatric community, as opposed to subgroups within the profession. Even the cover of *Archives*, which offered a list of articles, replicating the format of several other AMA journals, conveyed the message that psychiatry was moving back into the medical mainstream. From the beginning, *Archives* had a strong research agenda, even stronger than that of the *American Journal*.

When Grinker retired as editor in 1970, he was replaced by Daniel Xavier Freedman (1921–90), who held the position for the next twenty years. Danny Freedman played a crucial role in the transition to biological psychiatry. Trained as an analyst, Freedman was a diminutive but endlessly energetic man who served as chair of psychiatry at the University of Chicago from 1966 to 1984, at the time when Chicago became a great centre for biological research.

As his close friend Fred Goodwin told me, Freedman's first interest in psychiatry had been kindled as a teenager by reading Karl Menninger's book *The Human Mind.*[20] Freedman's training was at Yale, a bastion of analytic thinking. Like most bright young people who entered psychiatry after the Second World War, Freedman went through formal training at an analytic institute. But Freedman, who saw where the profession was heading, went on to become a researcher whose main contribution was as a leader and mentor.

Danny Freedman was a provocative and impish man, 'a scholar and a gadfly' (Goodwin), who knew everyone, and had influence both with the American Psychiatric Association and with members of Congress. His greatest impact on the field came through his editorship, at which he worked seven days a week. Goodwin sees the *Archives* as 'the child that Danny never had.'

Freedman had an uncanny judgment about submitted articles. Unlike other editors, he read all papers carefully, and his judgment was more important than formal peer review. Freedman always seemed to know when a paper would be a classic. When reviewers received articles to assess, Danny had already written comments all over them.

John Helzer of the University of Vermont, who had trained at Washington University, told me a typical story about Freedman.[21] Helzer had submitted a paper showing that when 'Research Diagnostic Criteria' (the precursors of DSM-III) are applied, psychiatric diagnosis can be as reliable as reading X-rays or electrocardiograms.[22] Seven reviews came back, all of them negative. Some were written by analysts who found the idea of making diagnoses based on algorithms rather disturbing. To them this kind of procedure undermined what analysis had brought to psychiatry: a recognition of the uniqueness of every patient. But Freedman ignored all the reviews, and published Helzer's paper as the leading article in the next issue of the *Archives.* It did indeed become a classic.

Freedman moved from Chicago to UCLA in 1984. He was so successful as editor of *Archives* that the AMA made the rare exception of allowing him to stay on after he turned sixty-five. Freedman died a few years later, still very much in the saddle.

Daniel Freedman was not a supporter of analysis, which found little or no space in the *Archives.* Yet Goodwin contrasts his views to those of other critics, who trivialized Freud's ideas only to discredit them. Freedman incorporated rather than dismissed the questions that analysis was designed to study. He believed that psychiatry would eventually have to answer the questions that Freud raised, but in an entirely different way. Goodwin agrees, suggesting that the most fruitful direction of future research will involve establishing links between brain activity and psychological phenomena.

How Analysts Became Biological Psychiatrists

Converts can be passionate about change, particularly when they enter new areas. Fred Goodwin remarks that the analysts who made the switch to biological psychiatry were 'more Catholic than the Pope.'

I have given examples in previous chapters of prominent psychiatrists who made this ideological shift. Robert Spitzer of Columbia was trained as an analyst, but allied himself with the fiercely anti-analytic group from Washington University. Spitzer went on to edit DSM-III, the diagnostic manual that eliminated all references to psychoanalytic theory. Allen Frances, another New York analyst, took virtually the same position when editing DSM-IV. I know Spitzer and Frances fairly well, since they have published research on personality disorders. Both have left psychoanalysis behind, and are fully converted to empiricism and pragmatism.

Herbert Pardes is a perfect example of the switch-over process. Trained in New York as a psychoanalyst, Pardes moved into research, became chair at the University of Colorado, headed NIMH, and then moved to Columbia, becoming both chair of psychiatry and dean of medicine. After his retirement from these positions, Pardes became CEO of a new merged hospital, New York Presbyterian (combining the teaching centres associated with Columbia and Cornell). I have heard Pardes lecture on many occasions, and he is a formidable speaker. One of his favourite topics is how developments in the neurosciences and genetics will shape the future of psychiatry. (I have never heard him say the same about psychoanalysis.)

It was not unusual in the 1960s for academic psychiatrists' offices to be routinely fitted with an analyst's couch. In my own hospital, couches were once regarded with awe as the tool of a powerful and arcane method of treatment. Over time, however, couches began to be used only as a convenient place for a quick nap. Another sign of the times is that I have sometimes seen them piled high with files and reprints. Most recently, I have even seen analytic couches used by nurses to give patients injections of antipsychotic medication.

A common pattern for analysts within academia is to avoid any formal break with the movement, but to place it at the periphery of one's professional life. John Gunderson is a good example. While completing his analytic training, he spent several years at NIMH as a researcher. Today

Gunderson is a full professor at Harvard and the doyen of research on borderline personality disorder. He remains sympathetic to psychoanalysis, and, along with Glen Gabbard and Peter Fonagy, has written an article calling for more research about its therapeutic efficacy.[24] But he identifies himself primarily as an academic psychiatrist.[25]

As I have found in my own career, conducting research changes one's ideas about treatment. Gunderson's views have evolved over the years: while his early work focused on how family problems were associated with the borderline personality, he later came to the conclusion that families who raise a child that has any serious disorder are, like the parents of schizophrenics, more victims than perpetrators. Gunderson has been conducting groups for some years with the families of patients, and has described psycho-educational methods to help them cope with their difficult children.[26] In his recent book on the clinical management of borderline personality, Gunderson presents a highly eclectic approach in which analytic therapy is only one of many elements.[27] His private practice is exclusively devoted to borderline patients, and he provides broad-spectrum therapy, only occasionally using the analytic couch.

Since analysts within academia are exposed to many different ideas, they usually become more eclectic in their practice than those whose professional contacts are limited to analytic institutes. At McGill's Department of Psychiatry, very few analysts on faculty see patients on the couch for more than a few hours a week, and several have abandoned analysis entirely. For one thing, the market is not there. Many patients clamoured for psychoanalysis thirty years ago. There was a mystique about the procedure, and analysts had waiting lists. One would even speak of one's predecessor in an analyst's schedule as having 'warmed the couch.'

Today analysis is mainly sought out by a small group of true believers. While troubled people still seek out therapy, and are often willing to pay for it, they are rarely interested in lying on a couch three or four times a week. For this reason, many analytically trained psychiatrists see patients once or twice a week, who sit in a chair facing the therapist.

One also no longer sees the kind of dramatic schisms in psychiatry between analysts and non-analysts that were prominent during my training. I can remember psychoanalysts thundering against biological treatments that they saw as sending patients down the drain. They were only a little less contemptuous of other psychological interventions, seeing behaviour therapy as simple-minded nonsense, and supportive therapy as little better than hand-holding. In the heyday of psychoanalysis, practitioners would stand up boldly on rounds, insisting that the patient under discussion absolutely *had* to be analysed. (If patients could not afford analysis, it was *their* responsibility, or their family's, to find the money.)

Today, analysts in academic settings are much more modest. They openly admit that their methods of treatment are not for everyone, and that only a small percentage of patients attending clinics can benefit from them. (As noted in chapter 5, this principle is openly acknowledged by the American Psychoanalytic Association.) Most analysts are reasonably up-to-date on psychopharmacology, and many are interested in rehabilitation psychiatry. They readily form alliances with colleagues with little interest or background in analytic therapy. For this reason, psychiatrists trained as analysts are not always recognizably different from their colleagues. I sometimes have had to ask around to find out who is an analyst and who is not.

Nonetheless, almost every major department of psychiatry in North America has members who remain committed to the analytic cause. At my own university, and at many others, they still form a constituency that no chair of psychiatry can ignore. Analysts are also faculty members who often win teaching awards from psychiatric residents. The reason is that they love to teach, and offer students a coherent theory and a model of humanistic treatment.

Researchers may be winning the 'glittering prizes' and rising to the top of the hierarchy. But they have little time to teach clinical psychiatry. A resident would not expect to be supervised on cases by famous researchers. By contrast, analytic supervisors will spend many hours teaching on a few cases, and are accordingly highly valued. They give residents in psychiatry the message that it is important to spend time talking to patients.

Most residents at top departments of psychiatry are not interested in research, and most graduates become clinical practitioners. As in previous generations, residents were attracted to psychiatry by a strong wish to understand and help people. While almost all accept evidence-based medicine in principle, they value 'hands-on' teachers who can explain (or seem to explain) what patients are telling them.

The Process of Transition at America's Top Medical Schools

Academic psychiatry has changed more through evolution than revolution. In chapter 2 I compared the varying histories and traditions at Harvard, Johns Hopkins, and Columbia. Today, these psychiatry departments, as well as most others that have a prominent role in North American psychiatry, look rather similar.

Harvard

The department at Harvard University remains decentralized, and is still spread over many sites. Its first official chair (appointed in 1990) was Joseph Coyle, a biological researcher who is now the editor of *Archives*. After Coyle stepped down, however, the teaching hospitals did not continue to support the position, and the Harvard department relapsed, having no one in charge.[28]

Yet all hospitals at Harvard today have a commitment to biological psychiatry. At Massachusetts Mental Health Center, where Elvin Semrad once reigned, the chief, until recently, was Ming Tsuang, a schizophrenia researcher and protégé of George Winokur at Iowa. At the Massachusetts General Hospital, psychoanalysis is almost invisible. At McLean Hospital, the once luxurious setting where long-term analytic treatment was a raison d'être, the standard stay for patients in the era of managed care is now five days, just long enough to be diagnosed and stabilized on drugs. To keep the hospital afloat, the directors have sold off half of the land and closed half the buildings. Nonetheless, McLean is still a jewel in the Harvard crown, with large biological laboratories and active psychosocial research.

Harvard has evolved, and must still be ranked as one of the top psychiatry departments in America. Research productivity at all sites remains high, and faculty who want to rise in the system must publish or perish. (Harvard's promotion process is notoriously strict.) The clinical teaching of psychotherapy to psychiatric residents continues to reflect analytic ideas. This may not be true in another ten or fifteen years. As older faculty retire, and as younger faculty are hired because of their research experience, Harvard might come to resemble departments in which analysis never held sway.

Johns Hopkins

Johns Hopkins University was never dominated by psychoanalysis, and its influence on the psychiatry department remains marginal. Paul McHugh, who served as chair for twenty-five years, retiring in 2001, was openly hostile to the movement, and was also a prominent and controversial opponent of the use of 'recovered memories' in psychotherapy.[29]

Johns Hopkins has been a centre for biological research, recruiting well-known investigators such as Solomon Snyder, a pioneer in the study of endorphins.[30] It gained some public notice for its special interest in sexual issues, although there have been some misadventures in that area. The department once sent patients for sex reassignment surgery (still a controversial procedure);[31] when it was noted that surgery failed to remove many psychological symptoms, the practice was discontinued. John Money, a Hopkins faculty member promoted the idea that gender identity was malleable in childhood,[32] but his ideas were contradicted by follow-up data (which became the basis of a best-selling book as well as of television programs).[33] As discussed earlier in this book, one cannot build medical science on clinical reports. Fortunately, science is self-correcting.

The new chair of the department, J. Raymond DePaulo, is a researcher on the genetics of mood disorders.[34] Johns Hopkins remains a leader in psychiatric epidemiology, and has conducted many important community surveys.[35] Overall, the department retains a standard of excellence that would make Adolf Meyer proud.

Columbia

This department is still one of the top psychiatric centres in the world. Its clinical operation, the New York State Psychiatric Institute, benefits from secure government funding. (Allen Frances, who worked briefly at Columbia, once described it as a virtual factory for the generation of grants.)[36] Under Governor Mario Cuomo, the state had agreed to fund a large new building for the Institute. When Cuomo was replaced by George Pataki, who originally had less interest in psychiatry, the plan was nearly cancelled.[37] Heinz Lehmann, then serving as deputy commissioner for mental health for the State of New York, was one of several people who helped change the governor's mind. In the end Pataki proudly attended the grand opening of the new Institute in 1999. Built on a bluff directly overlooking the Hudson River, the site commands a magnificent view and symbolizes the modernity of the department it houses.

The range of research interests at Columbia is impressive, and the department has great depth. Its most famous faculty member is Eric Kandel, the second psychiatrist in history to win a Nobel Prize. It also supports influential work on such topics as the neurobiology of suicide, medical genetics, and epidemiology. Until 2000, the chair of the department was Herbert Pardes, a former director of NIMH. While the search for his successor is still active (2004), it has focused on brain scientists, and thus Pardes may well have been the last psychoanalyst to serve as chair at Columbia.

Yale

Until the 1970s, New Haven was a great stronghold of psychoanalysis. While there was always biological research at Yale, from 1948 to 1967 the department was chaired by Fritz Redlich, a fairly orthodox analyst who had graduated from the University of Vienna in 1935. Redlich gained public attention with a book about Adolf Hitler,[36] but will probably be remembered best for showing that different social classes in New Haven receive different psychiatric treatment.[37]

Under Redlich, the atmosphere at Yale was favourable to analysis, so that psychiatrists like Theodore Lidz could flourish there. Lidz, whose textbook of child development was required reading during my residency, believed that pathological families are a main cause of schizophrenia.[38] For his book about the analytic treatment of psychosis,[39] Edward Dolnick interviewed Lidz, and described him as 'a lion in exile.' By the time Lidz died in 2001, he was a forgotten man.

In Redlich's time, the general hospital setting at Yale–New Haven Hospital was supplemented by the existence of the Yale Psychiatric Institute (YPI). Like McLean and Chestnut Lodge, YPI provided long-term care for adolescents and young adults with psychoses and personality disorders. Later, like the Menninger Clinic, it became a casualty of a changing *Zeitgeist* and of managed care. Tom McGlashan, an analyst who is a noted researcher on personality disorders and schizophrenia, was recruited from Chestnut Lodge in 1990 to run YPI. But the Institute was already in trouble. For a time, it had kept itself alive only by actively recruiting patients. (Some private hospitals in the United States even sent recruiters to find young people with substance abuse in Canada, since this was a time when some provincial governments provided unlimited benefits for treatment outside the country.) Like Chestnut Lodge and the Menninger Clinic, which went bankrupt and had to close, YPI also disappeared from the scene.

In 1969, Morton Reiser, another noted psychoanalyst, became chair at Yale. As Reiser told me,[40] this was a turbulent time on campus: on his first day on the job, he was locked in his office by hundreds of demonstrators. Reiser survived his baptism of fire, staying on until 1986, by which time analysis had begun to decline. A broad-minded man, Reiser has written about the need for intellectual rapprochement between psychoanalysis and psychiatry.[41] He has resisted radical critiques of analysis and believes that at least some of its theories can be reconciled with the data of neurobiological research. Yet it would be hard to find neuroscientists who would agree with that conclusion.

Reiser was first succeeded by Gary Tischler, a community psychiatrist, and then by Benjamin S. (Steve) Bunney, a biological researcher. Today, while the Yale department remains strong, analysts, as elsewhere, function as clinical teachers rather than academic leaders. Tom McGlashan is a good example of a psychoanalyst who 'made the switch.' After receiving research training at the NIMH, McGlashan never looked back. He conducted a long-term follow-up study at Chestnut Lodge that showed, among other things, that Fromm-Reichmann's much-vaunted treatment of schizophrenia had been ineffective.[42] Today McGlashan is involved with studies to identify young patients on the verge of psychosis.[43]

University of Chicago

The universities where analytic thinking flourished have tended to be in coastal locations, but every large city has had a large contingent of analysts. While Chicago has attracted famous psychoanalysts, from Franz Alexander to Heinz Kohut, the university department there has had a very different history

Psychiatry at the University of Chicago is located in a network of general hospitals that have been amalgamated. In the 1970s and 1980s, under the leadership of Danny Freedman, Chicago became a great centre for biological psychiatry, attracting stars like Herbert Meltzer, one of the doyens of neuropsychopharmacology. The next two chairs, Stuart Yudofsky (1990–2), a biological researcher, and Bennett Leventhal (1992–8), a child psychiatrist, were non-analysts. The current chair, Eliot Gershon, is one of the world's leading researchers on the genetics of mood disorders.[44]

Here, as we have seen elsewhere, analysts serve as clinical teachers but not as academic leaders; only one analyst is on full-time faculty. The Chicago Psychoanalytic Institute, the home base of Heinz Kohut, has little or no connection with the university. Eliot Gershon told me he was once invited to speak at the Institute, but felt very much like a visiting lecturer.[45] Since the University of Chicago was never dominated by analysis, it never needed a revolution.

University of California at San Francisco

Culturally, San Francisco resembles other large cities in which analysis has had a strong following. In the 1970s and early 1980s, Robert Wallerstein served as chair at the University of California at San Francisco (UCSF). He was a graduate of the Menninger Clinic and the author of a detailed book on the Menninger follow-up study.[46] Wallerstein is one of the most influential American analysts, and has served as a spokesman for the International Psychoanalytic Association, vigorously defending the discipline against its critics.[47] Thus, he was a typical departmental chair for his time; equally typical is the fact that analyst-chairs have almost entirely disappeared.

When Wallerstein stepped down, the dean of medicine wanted to make the department at UCSF a leader in biological psychiatry. The next chair was Sam Barondes (1986–96), a well-known researcher in the neurosciences; the current chair, Craig van Dyke, is also a biological investigator. As UCSF became a centre of research, analysis has taken a back seat, retaining its influence only through the clinical training program.

Charles Marmar is a Canadian psychiatrist who came to UCSF in 1976 to work with Mardi Horowitz, a psychoanalyst interested in the psychotherapy of post-traumatic disorders.[48] Horowitz's group at Mount Zion Hospital also tried to operationalize the key factors in psychoanalytic therapy, producing highly complex formulations (that were perhaps, in the end, more cognitive than Freudian). Marmar has retained his interest in trauma,[49] and is now one of America's leading experts on post-traumatic stress disorder (PTSD). But his research agenda long since left analysis behind.

Psychiatry at USCF is located in two general hospitals (San Francisco General and Mount Zion) and a psychiatric hospital (Langley Porter). As in most other universities, the psychoanalytic institutes in San Francisco have no formal links with UCSF. New faculty recruitments always focus on research, either in the neurosciences or in psychopathology. Moreover, the analytic institute, as elsewhere, split into several fragments based on ideological differences as well as on professional divisions between physicians and non-physicians. In the medical school, there is no money for research in psychoanalysis, and most academic psychiatrists tend to see the treatment as eclipsed by cognitive-behavioural and interpersonal therapy.[50] There is still a demand for formal analysis in the Bay area. As many as 20 per cent of UCSF graduates enter analytic training after their residency, and psychiatrists can earn a living in private practice.

University of California at Los Angeles

A unique factor in Los Angeles is the strong links between the analytic movement and Hollywood.[51] There is an enormous amount of money in the film community. Grateful patients have donated enormous sums to the university department. With additional strong financing from the state, UCLA has been in a position to attract academic stars like Danny Freedman.

The state of California, like New York, created a Neuropsychiatric Institute (NPI) for the study of mental illness that has been well funded. Phillip May's study showing that psychotherapy is ineffective for the treatment of acute psychosis was carried out at the NPI in the 1960s. Since then, the department has also had a Brain Institute for basic biological research in psychiatry.

From 1969 to 1989, the chair of the UCLA department was Louis Jolyon West (1923–99). Like many other leading psychiatrists of his generation, West came from a family of Russian Jewish immigrants (his mother gave him his unusual middle name after a character in Galsworthy's *The Forsyte Saga*).

'Joly,' as he was known to his colleagues, did not practise analysis, advocating instead a form of 'existential' therapy. Early in his career, he became known for describing the effects of brainwashing in the Korean War, and was known for his writings about cults.[52] West became a public figure when he testified for the defence at the trial of Patricia Hearst, where he argued that she should not be held responsible for her actions. (West also testified for the defence at the trial of Jack Ruby in 1964, while serving as chair of psychiatry at the University of Oklahoma.) West was a social activist who took strongly liberal positions, views that could have only made him more popular in Hollywood.

Jambur Ananth is an Indo-Canadian psychiatrist trained at McGill who was recruited to UCLA by West in 1980. According to Ananth, the chair could raise a million dollars in an evening simply by going out to dinner with a Hollywood luminary.[53] A charming man, West knew everyone who mattered in the film community. Although he knew little about biology, and was never a major researcher, West was the man who found the money to build the brain institute at UCLA.

The current chair of psychiatry at UCLA, Peter Whybrow, has a very different profile. Like his colleagues around North America, Whybrow has a neuroscience background and has studied the biology of mood disorders.[54] And as in other departments, analysts remain popular within their own sphere – clinical training. Jambur Ananth even wonders if psychotherapy is about to make a comeback in American psychiatry, as the marvels of psychopharmacology prove disappointing.[55] Yet residents at UCLA today are more likely to demand training in cognitive therapy. Over the last ten years, few have gone to either of southern California's analytic institutes, which now, like most others, mainly train candidates with backgrounds in psychology and social work.

Other American Universities

As psychiatry has moved into the mainstream, and as the coastal dominance of analysis declined, psychiatric departments in the American heartland have made their mark. Washington University in St Louis remains a great centre for research, and the University of Iowa, where George Winokur made such a powerful impact, continues to be productive, benefiting from strong support from the state government. The University of Pittsburgh, relatively unknown a few decades ago, given its record in obtaining grants, is considered by some to be number one in the country. (Like Harvard and Columbia, Pittsburgh has great depth, with research in many areas, from sleep disorders to schizophrenia.)

Psychiatric research has diffused to other prominent academic centres around the United States: in the South (e.g., Emory, Duke, and North Carolina), in California (e.g., UC San Diego and UC Davis), and the Midwest (e.g., Michigan and Wisconsin). None of the chairs of psychiatry at these universities are analysts. Being a psychoanalyst was once seen as a key qualification. Now it is at best an embarrassment, and at worst a liability.

The Canadian Scene

McGill University has always had a strong relationship between psychoanalysis and academic psychiatry. The first psychoanalytic institute in Canada was founded in Montreal,[56] where there is now an English and a French branch. Even today, some residents train at McGill because of its depth in analytic teaching.

The history of analysis at McGill can be charted through its academic leaders. The first chair of psychiatry at McGill, Ewen Cameron (1944–

63) was an eclectic trained at Maudsley and Johns Hopkins. He created a department in which every aspect of psychiatry was represented, and therefore encouraged the development of an institute by recruiting training analysts from England and the Continent. Cameron's successor, Bob Cleghorn (1963–70), was a trained analyst who was best known as a pioneer researcher in neuroendocrinology.[57] Heinz Lehmann (1970–4), Cleghorn's successor, was of course less sympathetic to analysis. He was followed by Maurice Dongier (1974–85), a French psychoanalyst. Like Cleghorn, Dongier practised analysis but maintained a much stronger commitment to research. The next chair, Gilbert Pinard (1986–96), was mainly interested in cognitive therapy. I have held this position since 1997.

Thus, at McGill, the pattern of academic leadership has paralleled what one sees south of the border. One cannot be a full professor or a chair without a strong research record. While analysts no longer dominate the teaching of psychotherapy as completely as they once did, they are still the most visible educators interested in talking therapies. At the same time, analysts continue to win teaching awards, and to have a strong influence on clinical training.

The story at the University of Toronto is quite similar. Toronto was the second city in Canada to have a psychoanalytic institute (opened in 1969), and it remains large and influential. In the past, analysts (Robin Hunter and Fred Lowy) have served as departmental chairs. In the last two decades of the century, however, the chairs at Toronto were Vivian Rakoff (1980–90), an adolescent psychiatrist known for theoretical scepticism,[58] and Paul Garfinkel (1990–2000), a noted researcher on eating disorders. The current chair, Don Wasylenki (2000–), is a trained psychoanalyst but is best known for research on the community treatment of schizophrenia.

Toronto, by far the largest psychiatric department in Canada, has benefited from the existence of a well-funded research hospital, the Clarke Institute (now, through a series of mergers, part of the Centre for Addiction and Mental Health). For many years, the psychotherapy service at the Clarke was led by analysts, who also dominated teaching at several other hospitals. Today, while psychoanalytic therapy continues to be taught, one of the unusual features at Toronto is its strength in non-analytic therapies. Over the last ten years, the leaders of the psychotherapy teaching program have been Molyn Lezcz,[59] a group therapist, followed by Zindel Segal,[60] a researcher in cognitive therapy.

This evolution may help to explain why Toronto graduates are practising differently after they complete residency. The department has conducted two unpublished surveys on practice, one in the early 1980s, and a second in the late 1990s.[61] Twenty years ago, psychiatrists were gravitating towards private practice consisting almost exclusively of long-term psychotherapy. (In Ontario, there are no limits on the length and frequency of sessions; even psychoanalysis is covered by provincial insurance.) Recently, graduates have generally developed hospital practices where they treat sicker patients and use much less psychotherapy. Economic factors do not account for this change; it probably reflects a shift in the residency program, in that young psychiatrists identify with different faculty members and learn a different set of skills.

Psychoanalysis in Canada largely remains a Montreal-Toronto phenomenon: 85 per cent of the analysts in Canada practise in one of these two cities.[62] (The United States has a similar pattern, with a majority practising in New York or Boston.) Even in the largest universities, the influence of psychoanalysis has receded. At the web site of the Canadian Psychoanalytic Society, Montreal analyst James Naiman describes the previous dominance of analysis in the universities located in Quebec and Ontario, and goes on to note, with obvious regret, 'At this writing no department of psychiatry in a Canadian medical school is headed by an analyst.'[63] (As noted above, there is now one exception, at Toronto.)

Other universities in central Canada, both French and English, have shown a similar evolution in the pattern of leadership. The University of Montreal has had several analyst-chairs in the past, and at one time the Institut Albert-Prévost (associated with Hôpital Sacré-Coeur), with strong links to the growing psychoanalytic movement in France, was a prominent centre for the application of analytic principles to psychosomatic medicine. Today, however, the university department is led by a non-analyst child psychiatrist, Sylvain Palardy, and none of the hospitals, including Sacré-Coeur, is dominated by analytic ideas.

Ottawa is one of only four cities in Canada (including two in Montreal and one in Toronto) that has opened its own analytic institute. (Elsewhere in Canada, anyone interested in analytic training has to travel.) A psychoanalyst (Gerald Sarwer-Forner) was chair of psychiatry at the University of Ottawa, but was replaced in 1985 by a psychopharmacologist (Yvon Lapierre), followed in 1995 by still another biological researcher (Jacques Bradwejn).

The department of psychiatry at McMaster University was founded, along with a new medical school, in 1967. The first chair was Nathan Epstein, a psychoanalyst trained in New York who had been chief of psychiatry at the Jewish General Hospital in Montreal. Epstein, a protégé of Nathan Ackermann, one of the pioneers of family therapy,[64] became interested in developing research methods to study this approach.[65] As he became increasingly committed to academic psychiatry, Epstein stopped believing in psychoanalysis, and eventually resigned from the society.[66] John Cleghorn, another psychoanalyst, was the next chair at McMaster, but he was an eclectic, with one foot in the neurosciences. As a medical school, McMaster became one of the most important centres in the world for evidence-based medicine. The psychiatry department has followed suit, and its most recent leaders (Russell Joffe and Richard Swinson) have been biological researchers.

Elsewhere in Canada, while some psychoanalysts are in practice, their influence in academia has been limited. Psychiatry in western Canada and the Maritimes has had many British-trained leaders, particularly from the Maudsley, and has therefore tended to be practical. Where psychoanalysis had no domain, there was no reason for a counterrevolution.

Part Three

DECLINE

chapter 7

The Future of Psychoanalysis

The Rise of Evidence-Based Medicine

For a long time, physicians had no standard for determining whether any of their treatments worked. Clinical practice depended not on empirical data but on the accumulation of experience. This is why bleeding and purging survived for centuries. While research on the causes of illness has often been scientific, medical practice has always remained more of an art. This gap has only recently started to narrow.

Evidence-Based Medicine (EBM)[1] advocates the application of quantitative, statistical, and empirical methods to determine whether treatment actually helps patients. (A similar movement has taken hold in clinical psychology, under the name of 'evidence-based practice.')[2]

In the past, medical practitioners considered it sufficient to publish a few case reports, or to describe percentages of success in a series of selected patients. Today, in the era of evidence-based medicine, all claims for therapeutic success must be tested systematically and published in peer-reviewed journals.[3] This principle lies at the centre of contemporary academic medicine.

Evidence-based medicine may seem commonsensical, but it is actually revolutionary. Instead of relying on authority and tradition, clinicians have become applied scientists. Psychiatric journals contain as much quantitative hard science as any other specialty.

The gold standard of EBM is the randomized controlled trial (RCT), the generally recognized standard for approving medical treatments.[4] In RCTs, effectiveness is determined by assigning patients randomly to different treatments (or no treatment), using measures of outcome that are 'blind' to the therapy that patients actually receive.

Physicians treating heart disease or cancer expect their interventions to meet the high standards required by RCTs. When they have been shown to be effective, expensive procedures such as cardiac surgery or bone-marrow transplants have been recommended by the profession and paid for by insurance.

Academic psychiatry has embraced EBM with enthusiasm. Departmental chairs and senior professors subscribe to the concept. At McGill, my reputation as an apostle and advocate for the movement has become a subject for local jokes. (When people disagree with a decision, they sometimes ask me whether I am practising evidence-based administration.) But the younger generation supports me. They understand that unless psychiatry becomes evidence-based, it will wither on the vine.

While cognitive-behaviour therapy has accepted and often met the standard of EBM,[5] psychoanalysis has not. The failure of analysis to become evidence-based has led to its becoming marginalized within academic psychiatry.

Yet many psychoanalysts are opposed to EBM.[6] They fear that an obsession with measurement has led physicians to forget how to be humane and caring. Analysts may also see EBM as nothing less than an attack on their practice and their world view. They have their own way of knowing, and their own kind of truth. (One also wonders whether some may be afraid of finding no proof for their therapeutic methods.)

There are also practical limitations to the value of EBM. Research is expensive, and many important issues in clinical practice have never been subjected to RCTs, and so clinicians are still dependent on accumulated experience. Another problem is, as Drew Westen has pointed out,[7] that patients who sign up for clinical trials are not typical of the complex cases physicians see in practice.

Still, the EBM movement is only at the beginning of a long process. Its methods will become more practical and sophisticated with time. While medical practice will always depend on skill and experience, physicians need to make decisions informed by evidence. For this reason, one can safely predict that, over the coming decades, EBM will have an increasing effect on clinical practice.

Does Psychoanalysis Work?

In its day, psychoanalysis was as avant-garde as a brain scan. Training in its methods was thought to provide access to the mind, a virtual X-ray of the unconscious. Psychoanalysis retained prestige in academic psychiatry as long as it was seen as a cutting-edge treatment.

The failure of psychoanalysis to meet these expectations was a crucial factor in its decline. Over and over again, I have heard analysts and former analysts describe the disillusionment they felt when promises were not kept. Whatever problems there are with theories, the bottom line about treatment is whether or not it works.

To give up a paradigm, one has to have an alternative. When belief is strong, there are always ways to reduce 'cognitive dissonance.'[8] For the therapist, one strategy is to take the position that change takes a long time. Then outcomes become impossible to measure, and you really cannot tell whether you have failed. Another strategy is to shift the paradigm. If older methods have failed, newer ones may succeed. Nonetheless, given the time and expense it requires, psychoanalysis needs to demonstrate at least some degree of unique efficacy. And even if it can be shown to work, does it work better than other methods?

As described in chapter 5, all talking therapies work through common mechanisms.[9] When analytic treatment has been compared to other methods, such as behaviour therapy,[10] it has shown no advantage. Even when analysis helps, results may emerge from applying non-specific factors such as a supportive relationship. It is even possible that psychoanalysis acts partly as a placebo (i.e., the expectation of improvement leads to real improvement).

The specific methods of psychoanalysis have never been shown to be uniquely effective. There is no empirical evidence that seeing patients longer, scheduling them more frequently, or putting them on a couch makes for any difference in outcome.[11] Nor is there anything magical about using the transference or in making interpretations. The research literature suggests that what therapists say does not make as much difference as how well patients feel understood.[12]

As early as the 1950s, in order to determine if there was something unique about the psychoanalytic method, the Menninger Clinic sponsored, at great expense, a classic study.[13] The project tried to answer questions about efficacy that, even then, were being raised by critics such as Hans Eysenck.[14] The Menninger researchers followed forty-two patients in formal analysis or psychoanalytic therapy. Unfortunately, there was no control group. Moreover, it took so long to collect the data that few of the original investigators were still at Menninger when the study was completed. The ultimate results were so confusing that the researchers almost gave up trying to make sense of them.

Otto Kernberg saved the day. Bringing in experts with advanced statistical knowledge to pull the study together, he became first author of a 'final report' published in 1972.[15] But the results of the Menninger study were disappointing. In spite of years of analysis, many patients continued to have serious difficulties. The main finding, that better-functioning people did better in therapy, has been described as only showing that 'the rich get richer and the poor get poorer.'[16]

A proper assessment of analytic therapy would have to meet contemporary standards for medical research, that is, an RCT. Physicians today are not expected to prescribe a drug on the basis of clinical impressions or uncertain data. In particular, they should not prescribe lengthy and arduous treatments until controlled trials prove that they really work.

Moreover, psychiatrists have judged psychoanalysis more as a treatment than as a theory. Thus, to bring analysis back into psychiatry, one would first have to prove the efficacy of analytic therapy, using the same standards as those developed for other methods. If psychoanalysis wants to be taken seriously, it has to play by these rules.

Donald Klein of Columbia[17] believes that psychoanalysis can be tested using the same procedures as any new drug presented for government approval.[18] The testing process would begin with a 'Phase I trial,' which determines if a treatment does harm. (This suggestion is not far-fetched: some patients get worse in psychotherapy.)[19] The next stage would be a 'Phase II trial,' systematically diagnosing a sample of patients as they enter analysis and obtaining outcome data using ratings from therapists, patients, and independent observers. Finally, psychoanalysis would be given a formal randomized controlled trial in a large sample. One would need to find patients willing to accept random assignment to a variety of treatments, including psychoanalysis, and make sure that the assessment of outcome was blind as to which form of therapy the patient was receiving. While this would be an expensive procedure, cognitive-behavioural therapy, as well as interpersonal therapy, have had their efficacy assessed according to this standard.[20]

This is very far from being the way analysis has been supported in the past. Most claims for the benefits of psychoanalysis have been based on clinical reports of success in individual cases. Present standards of evidence in medicine consider this kind of data next to useless. We cannot make inferences from single cases to larger clinical populations. We need empirical studies of large groups of patients (ideally, randomized controlled trials) to determine which, if any, patients should be referred for psychoanalysis.

If clinical trials are not conducted, then analysis will be further discredited. We lack evidence to show that psychoanalysis is more effective as a treatment than other methods, most of which are more cost-effective than spending years on the couch. These conclusions have been circulated in the media. Patients are voting with their feet, seeking out briefer and more focused methods of therapy.[21]

Thus, to get back into the game, psychoanalysis will have to do some serious research. I have heard many excuses over the years about how difficult the task would be. Yet this may only be a way for the movement to get itself off the hook. Even if it requires millions of dollars to conduct these studies, they must be carried out. And if NIMH does not come up with the money, the psychoanalytic movement should think about raising its own.

In 2002, three analyst-academics, Glen Gabbard, John Gunderson, and Peter Fonagy, published a leading article in the *Archives of General Psychiatry* entitled 'Retaining a place for psychoanalysis within psychiatry.'[22] The authors fully accepted the critique that analysis needs to prove its efficacy to remain part of medicine. They therefore proposed a large-scale clinical trial, in which analytic institutes around the world would require all their trainees supervised on cases to participate in a study. (This would not be a randomized controlled trial, but a 'naturalistic' study in which patients are followed over time to see whether or not they improve.)

Robert Michels, an analyst who is a professor at Cornell, sees this idea as impractical, given that it would require cooperation from institutes that are inherently hostile to research.[23] Instead, he argues, it would be better to conduct a multi-site research project at several universities. Initial funds might come from private donations (wealthy ex-analysands). At McGill University, a group of researchers led by a psychiatrist, Chris Perry, are hoping to carry out this kind of clinical trial. Perry, who says that 'psychoanalysis has not had its day in court,'[24] is determined to put the method to the test. He proposes to randomly assign a large group of patients with chronic symptoms to psychoanalysis, long-term analytically oriented psychotherapy, long-term CBT, and supportive therapy. It remains to be seen whether he can carry through such an elaborate and expensive study.

Why is it that these proposals, so noble in intention, are difficult to fund? The reason is that today psychoanalysis is too far outside the research *Zeitgeist* – even mentioning analytic theory in a grant application can be as good as poison. Yet it is no longer enough to call for research as a way of fending off criticism. After one hundred years of analytic practice with no supporting data, someone has to carry out this task.

Clinical Tales and Fables

Therapists like to write about therapy. But they do not always tell the truth. The facts are that while some patients get remarkably better, others entirely fail to respond. The majority are helped and comforted without being cured.

Since the time of Freud, the efficacy of psychoanalysis has been supported by case histories. Yet I have always thought there was something suspicious about them. The clinical tales I read in journals and books are often fables with happy endings. Evidently, people get remarkably better as soon as therapists help them to achieve some crucial insight. From the tales I have read, one gets the impression that it is not unusual to receive a slice of wedding cake at the end of treatment.

When I started to write up some of my own cases, I was also tempted to gild the lily. No one wants to admit failure, and no one wants to hear about failure, even if that is the simple truth. Books on therapy sell because they offer hope. Conferences featuring lectures by famous therapists are popular for the same reason. Like revival meetings, they are inspirational events designed to raise the spirits of frustrated clinicians.

Consider the following example. Twenty-five years ago, I attended a talk by a psychoanalyst who had authored a best-selling account of his treatment of a New York call girl.[25] As a medical student I had read this book, which was one of several that made me want to become a therapist. According to the published account, treatment was successful. After understanding the impact of her traumatic childhood, the patient found a good man who loved her, and gave up her unsavoury life.

After hearing the author lecture, I asked him if he had recent news from his former patient. He grimaced and told me that he indeed hears from her regularly, and that her life is one of uninterrupted loneliness and misery. When I suggested that the author should consider publishing a second edition of his book containing this information, he did not respond.

This story illustrates the importance of following up on one's cases. To assess the results of treatment, outcome needs to be documented over time. I became interested in this problem over twenty years ago after developing a special clinical interest in suicidal patients with borderline personality disorder. Many of these cases had been admitted to a hospital unit where patients often spent months receiving intensive analytic therapy. Afterwards, they disappeared from the system. What happened to them? Were they cured? Were they still alive?

My research team eventually located one hundred former patients after an average of fifteen years.[26] (Twelve years later, we located most of them again for a twenty-seven-year follow-up.)[27] Although 10 per cent eventually died by suicide, most of the 90 per cent who were alive had greatly improved. But it had taken ten to fifteen years for these patients to recover. Surprisingly, those who received little therapy seemed to do just as well as those who spent years in treatment.

Some patients get better as they grow older, independent of treatment. This is a well-known phenomenon among substance abusers and criminals, most of whom, if they survive, improve by middle age.[28] This natural recovery over time helps to create the illusion that long therapies are necessary. Time is the healer, but the analyst gets the credit.

All the same, even after months to years of hard work, many patients fail to get better. Moreover, all psychiatrists know stories of patients who, after being in analysis for years with no visible results, eventually improved after receiving antidepressants. This scenario has been discussed in books and in the media;[29] as the public has learned about the effects of drugs, it has lost confidence in the value of analysis.

Psychoanalysts, who are ingenious at explaining so many things, are also creative in accounting for failure. One of the most frequent arguments one hears is that the treatment has not lasted long enough. This is probably why patients can stay on the couch for as long as fifteen years. In his old age, Freud himself was disappointed in the results of analysis.[30] Many patients continue treatment out of hope and habit, and only abandon it when either they, or the analyst, move away or die.

In a psychiatry building, I often saw a rich woman with fine clothes and an expensive coiffure. She must have had hardly any life outside, since she spent so many hours chatting up secretaries and receptionists. She was treated for over thirty years, and her analyst stated that therapy would only terminate when one of them died. As it turned out, he was the one to die first. The patient, who could easily afford it, went on to seek more treatment from another analyst. Recently, a colleague of mine ran into her, and found her much improved – her new therapist had prescribed antidepressants.

True Believers and Fellow Travellers

The dominance of psychoanalysis in academic psychiatry did not depend only on faculty who were formally trained analysts. Many psychiatrists who practised psychotherapy were sympathizers and fellow-travellers of the analytic movement. I was one, and so were many of my colleagues. Most of us had been through personal analysis. Moreover, the ethos of our community was that one should go *back* into analysis (for a 'retread') whenever new problems arose in life. One survey of psychotherapists showed that the majority have multiple experiences as patients in therapy over the course of their lifetime.[31] Early in my residency, when I mentioned to a teacher that I was in analysis, he asked, 'What, only the first one?'

The ubiquity of personal analysis created special problems. You had to know who was in analysis with whom. Otherwise, you might say something nasty about a senior teacher that could be reported back to that person the next day. In such an environment, voicing criticism within the hearing of a colleague could be dangerous. Even as a department chair, I have to take into account the possibility that members of my faculty currently in analysis may be talking about me on the couch, and getting support for their complaints.

Many forces worked to make psychotherapists in academic psychiatry form a tightly knit community. We attended rounds led by senior analysts. We created small groups for peer supervision in which we commented on each other's cases, always from a psychoanalytic perspective. Unlike the young psychiatrists of today, who tend to work full-time in hospitals, we spent half of our week conducting long-term therapy. Although I was never a true believer, the treatment model I used in my practice and taught to my students was essentially psychoanalysis. After a few weeks of supervision, one of my residents said to me, 'You're some kind of neo-Freudian, aren't you?' I had to acknowledge he was more or less on the mark.

Personality disorders became the focus of my career – as a clinician, as an educator, and a researcher. For this, I have to thank my psychoanalytic supervisors who were interested in this problem. Initially, loyal to Heinz Lehmann, I saw these patients as suffering from chronic depression. But once I began to diagnose them with borderline personality disorder, I had a much better frame for understanding them. Sometimes the patients helped me out. One day, a man with whom I was having endless problems walked into the office, and handed me a reprint of an article by Otto Kernberg on borderline personality, saying, 'Read this – it might help.'

Working with chronically suicidal patients was exciting, since it drew on my medical background as well as my psychotherapy training. Therapy turned on life-or-death issues At the very least, I could determine the outcome: the patient would either be alive or dead.

My special interest in this difficult population did not mean I had a secret formula for successful therapy. I did not even have a good theoretical model. I had been trained to believe that personality disorders were mainly the result of an unhappy childhood. Therefore, the job of the therapist was to discover these connections and explain them to the patient. Relationships between past and present problems in a patient's life create what psychiatrists call a 'psychodynamic formulation.'[32] In this exercise, current conflicts are understood as a reaction to and repetition of past events.

As a young faculty member, I quickly became a master of the formulation game. It was tempting to demonstrate my virtuosity to students, impressing them, much as I had been impressed by my own teachers. Over time, however, I began to wonder if being clever was the same as being right. It is all too easy to find childhood traumas in people's histories. I could probably pick anyone off the street, with or without symptoms, and pinpoint a few. Analytic theory also had fudge factors (such as repression and denial) to account for troubled patients who stubbornly insisted that their childhood had been happy.

While my formulations were glib, and my students loved them, when I presented them to patients, nothing magical happened. A typical interpretation might go something like this: 'You are doing the same thing with your boyfriend and your boss that you did with your mother when you were a child. You adapt to their needs and ignore your own, and in the long run that only makes you angry and depressed.' Assuming the comment was reasonably on target, patients might agree. Yet such interventions, by themselves, rarely lead to change.

Psychoanalysis adds another twist – the transference. Thus, in the above example, one might add: 'I also notice you do the same with me. You say it doesn't matter if I'm a few minutes late, but every time that happens you clam up afterwards.' These 'complete interpretations'[33] (links between present, past, and transference) are supposed to be uniquely effective. David Malan believed that they could also be used in brief analytic therapy.[34]

But research has not supported the unique value of interpretations in therapy. At best, analytic therapy goes better when the therapist establishes a clear theme and follows it consistently during the session.[35] Many analysts acknowledge that interpretations do not produce short-term results, but emphasize that learning takes time. It has been said that it take weeks to understand patients, but years to change them.

While Freud's treatments took months, the average analysis today

lasts for many years.[36] The extreme length of treatment can be rational-
ized in various ways. One reason given is that patients may need to make
the same mistakes over and over again before they can change. The task
of the analyst is to say, as Ronald Reagan famously said to Jimmy Carter
in their 1980 debate, 'There you go again.' Yet patience can provide a
convenient excuse for stasis and failure. Analyses can become endless
when they are not working and no one wants to admit it.

Lies My Fathers Told Me

After years of experience as an analytically oriented therapist, I could
not avoid noticing that my results were at best middling. Like everyone
else, I had a few triumphs. (These are the cases therapists like to talk
about.) I also had patients who failed to improve, and a few who got
worse. Most fell between these extremes.

Was I that much worse than other therapists? Surely, I thought, my
colleagues down the hall must be doing better. But I heard about their
cases in conferences and rounds: everyone else was having the same
trouble I was, and with the same kind of patients. Did the analysts know
more than I did? When I talked to colleagues who had been in treatment with local training analysts, I was not so sure. Psychoanalysts talk a
good game, but don't always come through with the goods.

In the early years of my practice, I attended many conferences and
lectures given by senior clinician-analysts, hoping to imbibe their wisdom. The speakers were often charismatic, but their ideas rarely helped.
Then I tried devouring the library. Some analysts wrote well and
described their work in detail, while others were so lost in theoretical
formulations that one wondered if the author had ever seen a patient.
Even so, how could I know whether their methods would be effective in
my hands? When, under the influence of Robert Langs,[37] I tried to
focus every therapy session on transference issues, a patient brought me
up short: 'What makes you think that everything I say has to do with the
way I feel about you?'

Around this time, I was treating a young woman who had made a serious suicide attempt. Alarmed by the situation, I obtained two consultations from senior psychoanalysts. To their credit, neither suggested that
I had failed to make the right interpretations. By now, the conventional
wisdom of analysis had changed, and more emphasis was being placed
on creating a healing relationship. The first consultant, Henry Kravitz,
advised me that I needed to enjoy seeing the patient (I did not). The

second consultant, who had studied under Elvin Semrad in Boston, quoted his old teacher as saying, 'When you're in trouble with a patient, don't lean back, lean forward.' These consultations were of little practical help, but they calmed me down for a while. My patient eventually did well, though I will never know whether this happened because of, or in spite of, the therapy.

I eventually stopped worrying about making correct interpretations to patients. For a time, like a priest who had lost his faith, I continued to say mass, but the words were empty. Gradually, I learned to set my sights lower, and to accept that I was treating patients with chronic illnesses, and there would be no miracles. After years of experience, most therapists come to similar conclusions. One either lowers one's expectations or gets out of the field.

Why hadn't my teachers told me this? The fact that they had not made me think of a film title from the 1970s, *Lies My Father Told Me*. And why didn't famous therapists, the authors of the books I had been reading, freely admit their limitations? Were they only lying to their readers, or were they also hiding the truth from themselves by telling fairy tales about therapeutic success?

Ultimately, my disillusionment about the results of long-term therapy turned into a positive experience. I no longer felt inadequate and frustrated, but was happy to achieve small gains for troubled people. I also became a different kind of teacher. I gave up reproducing my own education, and stopped offering glib remedies. I now tell my students the truth: psychiatrists don't always understand mental illness very well, but they can still help people.

I am reminded of another scene from the cinema. In a film from the 1970s, *Blume in Love*, a patient asks her psychiatrist why he practises therapy when he doesn't know whether it works or not. He replies, 'This is what we have to do until we find something better.'

Myths of Childhood

Psychoanalysts were the pioneer theorists of child development. Many of the early-childhood psychiatrists had an analytical training. Yet today, the ideas of Freud about childhood, or later theories developed by Erik Erikson[38] and Melanie Klein,[39] have become anachronistic. The *only* psychoanalytic idea about childhood that is taken seriously today in the scientific community is John Bowlby's attachment theory.[40]

Quietly but firmly, most analysts have long since discarded the Freudian apparatus of ego, id, and superego. Few consider the Oedipus complex to be of great importance. What then makes psychoanalysis a unique theory?

The last bastion of Freud's thought is the existence of an *unconscious.* Few scientists doubt the existence of an unconscious mind.[41] But it cannot be assessed through clinical observation. Analysts who believe their method provides access to unconscious thoughts are fooling themselves. As Adolf Grunbaum pointed out in an influential book,[42] Freud's ideas about the meaning of free associations, dreams, and neurotic symptoms were just as likely to be determined by his own preconceptions as by his patients' unconscious.

Science has also questioned the precise impact of childhood experiences. This is another idea central to Freud's thought, at the core of analytic therapy. Everything is geared towards explaining the present through the past. Trained by analysts, I always took it for granted that these parallels are deeply meaningful. However, seeing large numbers of patients changed my mind.

Over the last thirty years, I have run a teaching clinic that evaluates hundreds of new patients a year. Over thirty years, I have carried out thousands of consultations. (When my residents express surprise at my ability to recognize patterns quickly, I tell them their assessments will also get better after the first 10,000 cases.)

These experiences gave me a different perspective on the impact of childhood. Many patients report childhood adversities and trauma. Yet, if one keeps an open mind, one observes others with the same symptoms who report nothing unusual about their early life. Moreover, patients with minor problems can report the same childhood experiences as those with severe problems.

The impact of adversity depends on the individual. Research strongly confirms this conclusion. For example, only 20 per cent of people who have been sexually abused as children experience serious problems later in life.[43] People with terrible childhoods can turn out to be normal adults, and some people with serious problems have had a normal childhood.

So how did psychiatrists get this wrong? Again, one can easily be fooled by preconceptions. Our data base is limited to clinical experiences with troubled patients, many of whom are all too happy to blame their families for their problems.

Childhood is not easy for everyone. Yet early experiences do not necessarily provide an adequate explanation for adult symptoms. When I wrote a book on this subject a few years ago,[44] I received comments on my draft from Judith Rich Harris, author of the best-selling volume, *The Nurture Assumption*.[45] In her book, Harris had argued that parents are not necessarily the most important factor in a child's life. She found it almost unbelievable that a *psychiatrist* agreed with her.

Michael Rutter, the acknowledged dean of child psychiatry in Britain, and one of psychiatry's greatest thinkers, came to similar conclusions.[46] Sir Michael (or Mike, as he prefers to be addressed) is an owlish man with an unassuming manner who has spent most of his life working at the Maudsley Hospital, the great psychiatric hospital on the south bank of the Thames.

I have learned to cherish the way British people think. They have fewer enthusiasms than Americans, but tend to be more commonsensical. To be fair, Britain has had its own share of analytic zealots, from Melanie Klein to R.D. Laing. John Bowlby probably represented British culture at its best. Taking nothing for granted, he was always ready to change his mind when the evidence pointed another way. (It may not be an accident that Bowlby's last book was a biography of Charles Darwin.)[47] Michael Rutter is cut from the same cloth. Trained in research methodology, he has devoted his career to sorting out the factors that determine what kind of adults children grow up to be. The real story is much more complex than in the Freudian version.

Since Freud, analysts have been telling dramatic tales about the life-long consequences of childhood events. Most people prefer simple explanations, and these ideas are appealing. When one reads Rutter, the poetic certainties of analytic writing are replaced by paragraphs listing six or seven different factors that could determine the outcome of anyone's childhood experience.

The true course of human life is complex and chaotic. No connections can be taken for granted and nothing in development is straightforward. When I took a course with Rutter, a student asked him why he never referred to the developmental sequences proposed by Freud and Erikson. Rutter's reply was that he had always been suspicious of grand theories that usually have little scientific evidence behind them.

If childhood events do not really determine adult life, then most of what analysts have been telling their patients is either wrong or vastly oversimplified. As Jeffrey Masson once quipped in a different context,[48] analysts may have to announce the biggest recall since the Ford Pinto.

The history of child psychiatry reflects this sea change in theoretical thinking. In the universities where analysis dominated, child psychiatry was virtually a branch of psychoanalysis. Today, the leaders of academic child psychiatry are scientists. Child psychiatrists have also been leaders in community psychiatry and the development of multi-disciplinary teams. To see how much the field has changed, one only needs to open the leading periodical in the field (the *Journal of the American Academy of Child and Adolescent Psychiatry*, often called 'The Orange Journal'). In its pages, one can readily see that analysis is absent, having been replaced by empirical research on topics ranging from epidemiology to neurobiology.

The Attack on Psychoanalysis

In 1975, Peter Medawar (1915–87), a world-famous medical researcher in immunology, wrote an article in the *New York Review of Books* that concluded: '[T]he opinion is gaining ground that doctrinaire psychoanalytic theory is the most stupendous intellectual confidence trick of the twentieth century, and a terminal product as well – something akin to a dinosaur or a zeppelin in the history of ideas, a vast structure of radically unsound design and with no posterity.'[49]

But while the dinosaur has suffered many wounds, it is far from extinct. In spite of its failure to prove its effectiveness, psychoanalysis continues to be practised. In spite of its failure to become a science, analytic theory is still being taught to psychiatrists. While analysis is no longer dominant in academic psychiatry, it is still a constituency that cannot be ignored. Perhaps the survival of psychoanalysis simply reflects a time lag, as an older generation dies off and a younger generation comes to maturity.

One of the most devastating attacks on psychoanalysis came from the Harvard psychiatrist Alan Stone, who concluded that its only future lies as a tool for literary analysis.[50] (Given the present state of literary criticism, this may not have been a compliment.) Actually, the tendency for psychoanalysis to be more important in the intellectual culture than in medicine is not new. Yet when psychoanalysis starts to lose support from *outside* the scientific community, it needs to be particularly concerned.

In 1995, the *New York Review of Books* published a series of stinging articles by Frederick Crews, an English professor who had once been a strong sympathizer of analysis, and then turned into a ferocious opponent.[51] (It is telling that the *New York Review*, an important intellectual opinion-maker, has published critics like Medawar and Crews.) Psychoanalysts were deeply wounded by Crews's comments, which produced a

large body of correspondence to the *New York Review*. The Chicago analyst Marian Tolpin wrote that Crews's imperative was 'to pronounce all
of contemporary psychoanalysis worthless and/or destructive.'[52]

These howls of outrage occurred in response to a radically changed
world. When everyone believed that psychoanalysis was the ultimate
form of psychotherapy, its practitioners were lionized by the media, and
asked to pontificate on almost any subject.

What the public is more likely to hear today concerns the question 'Is
Freud Dead?' (This was the title of a *Time* cover story from 1993,[53] illustrated with a picture of Freud, showing his image cracking and peeling.)
When the Library of Congress organized an exhibition on Freud in 1996,
a controversy emerged.[54] In its original form, the exhibit had presented
an idealized picture of the man and his work – the standard view of Freud
as a prophet and seer. Protests from critics (such as Crews) led to a post-
ponement of the exhibit, which, when it eventually opened in 1998,
acknowledged the continuing disputes about Freud's ultimate impact.

Analysts talk about the modernity of contemporary analysis,[55] and call
their opponents 'Freud bashers,' complaining that criticism has been
hostile and indiscriminate.[56] Analysts also like to emphasize how far they
have moved beyond their founder. The message is 'Don't criticize
Freud. We've come a long way since.' In the view of the defenders of
analysis, the recent barrage of criticism runs the risk of throwing out the
baby with the bathwater. But the challenges to psychoanalysis have been
so far reaching that one wonders whether there will be a baby left when
the bathwater is drained.

How Psychoanalysts Have Responded to Criticism

The psychoanalytic movement has responded to criticism in four ways:
fundamentalism, revisionism, demedicalization, and *the flight from treatment.*

Fundamentalism

I regularly check out the *Journal of the American Psychoanalytic Association*
and the *International Journal of Psychoanalysis*. For all the talk about the
modernity of contemporary analysis, to judge from the papers in these
standard journals, the field has not evolved. Most of what is being published could just as well have appeared fifty years ago. As we have seen,
this is not the case for the *American Journal of Psychiatry*. For analysis,
however, nothing essential has changed.

The fundamentalist point of view was mainstream for the old guard, and it has even had some appeal for psychiatrists of my own generation. One training analyst I know no longer even considers himself a psychiatrist – as I found out when I introduced him at a lecture, and he insisted on being identified *only* as a psychoanalyst. Analysts who take a fundamentalist position usually have office practices, and work only part-time in academia. At the Montreal institute, I watched Drew Westen being criticized simply for saying that psychoanalysis has to be revised to be consistent with current psychological research.

No analyst would ever admit to being a fundamentalist. Everyone claims to be modern in one way or other. If one had to look for an example of a true believer, it might come from the New York Psychoanalytic Institute, where Charles Brenner still works: his book on psychoanalytic theory was assigned reading for me as an undergraduate in 1958, and is still used as an educational tool.[57]

Ultimately, fundamentalism in psychoanalysis is unlikely to endure. Fidelity to Freud does not inspire a younger generation who are less hostile to the scientific method.

Revisionism

Revisionists aim to save psychoanalysis by changing it. They accept the need to rebuild the model on an empirical base and to prove that treatment really works. They take more interest in the social context of suffering, and can be skilled in group and family therapy. Some have learned to use drugs effectively in conjunction with psychoanalysis.

Most analysts within the academic community can be described as revisionists. I have discussed the work of several of them: among the best and brightest are Peter Fonagy, Glen Gabbard, and Drew Westen. These people do not see psychoanalysis as a Zeppelin, but as an older yet still serviceable craft that can still get you where you want to go.

Yet patching up psychoanalysis may not work. Turning analysis into a science will require a much more radical revision. Any new model will have to be in accord with developments in psychology and the neurosciences. The result may well be unrecognizable as psychoanalysis.

Demedicalization

Freud did not think that psychoanalysis had to be tied to medicine.[58] His view reflected his resentment towards mainstream psychiatrists who rejected his ideas. Few psychoanalysts have a serious scientific training. This was true even when most were MDs. Physicians are expected to know *something* about science, but most have little direct experience with empirical methods. While the admission of PhD psychologists to analytic institutes might have addressed this problem, a PhD is no guarantee of a rigorous scientific training.[59] Then, as psychiatrists stopped applying to analytic institutes, training was opened to candidates from a wide range of professional backgrounds, including the humanities. This trend follows the tendency for analysis to move away from medicine and become more of a philosophy or a way of life. I have known psychoanalysts who come from backgrounds that are far from medicine and psychology: English professors, business professors, and political-science professors. One gets the impression that Alan Stone was right, and that psychoanalysis is now closer to the humanities than to medicine.

The Flight from Treatment

Some analysts have rejected the relevance of scientific inquiry. A 'hermeneutic' or 'postmodern' epistemology has a certain cachet in the humanities.[60] In this view, there is no such thing as objective truth. Thus, what patients tell analysts is more like a literary text than a piece of data. What analysts tell their patients would be only one of many possible interpretations.[61]

Denying the existence of objective truth is a tempting position for a discipline that has been unable to establish solid standards of evidence. These ideas might also appeal to the same people who think that shamans are just as good as physicians. It doesn't matter what the truth is, as long you make up a good story. Needless to say, accepting postmodernism in this way would sound the death knell for analysis within psychiatry. If psychoanalysis is to be nothing more than a narrative or a commentary on a text, it can not be credible either as a method of healing or as a science.

Some practitioners have gone so far as to redefine psychoanalysis as something other than a treatment. Being analysed can be seen as either an end in itself or a creative venture. Analysts who take this view do not promise patients that they will be cured of symptoms. Maurice Dongier, a former chair of psychiatry at McGill, has said that analysis is a creative exploration that provides insight but not cure.[62]

None of these responses is really adequate. Fundamentalism is not an option, since it would only deepen the gap with academia, and would probably turn off most of its current practitioners. Revisionism has a long way to go if it hopes to preserve the core of analysis while modernizing it. Analysis can not be postmodernist without separating itself entirely from medicine. Defining psychoanalysis as something other than treatment can only hasten its demise. The only stance that has any hope for retaining a place for psychoanalysis within psychiatry would be a rapprochement with science.

Can Psychoanalysis Be Reconciled with Science?

The problem with psychoanalysis is not that it is too complicated, but that it is too simple. As a theory, it is no longer compatible with current ideas in cognitive and developmental psychology. Attempts to revise psychoanalysis in the light of current scientific knowledge have been slow and grudging. As a therapy, its failures were rooted in grandiose claims, unsupported by data. This is why it lost so much ground to cognitive-behaviour therapy, which built in research from the very beginning.

One important caveat should be registered here. While CBT has documented its effectiveness in many conditions, it is no more a panacea than is psychoanalysis. Some of its practitioners can be as messianic as analysts. In fact, we have a long way to go in developing efficacious psychological treatments. Interestingly, as cognitive-behavioural therapists have been taking on more difficult patients, they have developed models that use some of the concepts of psychoanalysis, such as transference and resistance.[63] One wonders if CBT will run into the same problems of excessive treatment length and long-term support that have plagued psychoanalytic therapy.

A convergent process is taking place in psychoanalysis. Many analysts today see patients once or twice a week in sitting-up 'psychodynamic therapy' rather than formal, three-to-four-times-a-week analysis. In the real world, many analysts are less silent, make more active interventions, and are more practical in their approach to patients. The differences between analysis and CBT are much less striking than they used to be.

Eventually, psychotherapy will develop into a single discipline bringing together many theoretical perspectives. One will not have to ask the therapist one sees what kind of approach will be used; it will be sufficient if clinicians are properly trained and licensed. Therapists in the future will probably spend less time talking about patients' childhood experiences. We can conclude from the success of non-analytic forms of therapy that most people get better, not by spending years remembering their past, but by changing their behaviour in the present.

Robert Michels, an analyst-academician, trained at the National Institute of Mental Health in the 1960s. After returning to New York, Michels served as chair of psychiatry and dean of medicine at Cornell, and is associated with the psychoanalytic institute at Columbia University, where he still teaches. Michels has come to the conclusion that establishing strong links to the sciences is the only hope for psychoanalysis.[64] Like many others, he fears that psychiatry could become another medical specialty that values technology over people, and that its practitioners may stop talking to patients. At the same time, Michels criticizes psychoanalysis for not developing a methodology that can lead to progress. He points out that science has a cumulative, additive, and progressive quality. Yet while analysts sometimes come up with new ideas, the discipline has never developed a way to discard old ideas, an essential feature of scientific progress.

Michels has little hope that the leaders of psychoanalysis will join scientific medicine. They *know* their treatment works and only want to convince others. This attitude is contrary to science, where one always has to be ready to discard pet theories in the face of new evidence. The leaders of psychoanalysis are practitioners, not researchers. They grew up in a world where the ambition was to teach, not to investigate. The most prestigious members of the institutes are the training analysts, some of whom go on to become presidents of national and international associations. At universities, by contrast, promotion depends on conducting research. Moreover, since institutes do not get enough candidates from medicine, they have moved away from psychiatry. In Michels's view, they are trade schools that exist to market analysis, not to study it. Research will have to come from the academic culture, and the first area to be evaluated should be analytic treatment.

Other thoughtful analysts have come to similar conclusions. Drew Westen, a researcher who obtained an analytic training, published a review article on links between the field and empirical data in the prestigious journal *Psychological Bulletin*.[65] Glen Gabbard and Peter Fonagy are very much 'on the same page.'

The problem is that research in the neurosciences has not really provided support for psychoanalytic theory. While some psychoanalysts have made claims that studies of brain reward systems confirm the ideas of Freud,[66] this connection is quite a stretch. It is much more likely that research in the neurosciences will lead to an entirely new theory of the mind, rather than resurrect one that is a hundred years old.

We do know more about systems in the brain that modulate key psychopathological phenomena.[67] It has even been shown that successful psychotherapy produces measurable brain changes.[68] Yet none of these findings shows that science has confirmed the essence of analytic theory. This is not really surprising, since psychoanalysis was extrapolated from clinical data, as opposed to being based on systematic observations.

The claim that psychoanalysis is itself a science derives from a time when anybody with an interesting theory could claim to be a 'scientist.' (Karl Marx called his system 'scientific socialism.') While philosophers still argue about the precise boundaries of science, however, there is a consensus about its essence: *hypotheses must be tested with measurable data.*[69] No theory of the mind, and no method of treating patients, can survive without empirical testing.

While these principles are generally accepted, it is difficult to practise psychiatry entirely on the basis of scientific data. One of the attractions of psychoanalysis has always been that it offers a coherent theory of mind. The question is whether psychiatry is better off with an inadequate theory, or with none at all. Perhaps we simply need to be patient, and wait until there is enough data to support a coherent theoretical model of the mind.

The most lasting legacy of psychoanalysis is likely to be its humanism. The analytic approach encourages therapists to listen to and understand troubled patients. The question is whether its theories help or impede the process of empathy.

Theories have always been important in medicine. Without Harvey's physiology of circulation, cardiology would be unthinkable. Even in psychiatry, the action of drugs has been partially explained by theories about brain chemistry. But these models have had to survive rigorous testing. It is no longer acceptable to speculate about the unconscious or about the effects of childhood experience on adult life. These ideas have to be turned into measures that researchers can use with precision.

The most basic elements of Freud's model were the existence of an unconscious mind and the childhood origins of psychological problems. As we have seen, research findings have challenged both of these elements. While unconscious processes undoubtedly exist, they may not take a form that Freud would recognize. Nor does the existence of an unconscious mind prove the validity of psychoanalysis, since the concept is just as basic to cognitive theory. As Horatio said to an equivocating Hamlet, 'There needs no ghost, my lord, come from the grave to tell us this.'

Similarly, while adult psychological problems are influenced by events during childhood, the relationship is unpredictable and weak. Current stressors and underlying temperament are better predictors of whether people are mentally healthy and develop adverse psychological symptoms. Science has not shown that development during childhood has any particular sequence or confirmed the effects of early experience on adult life described by Freud and his followers.

In the academic world, you are not allowed to indulge yourself with too many theoretical speculations. You have to get out and test your ideas. If, as seems to be the case with psychoanalysis, the theory is too complicated to test, you are best advised to throw it out and work out a simpler one. These are the rules in psychology, and they are also the rules in medicine. If analysts want to be taken seriously in science, they will have to play the same game as everyone else.

The Legacy of Psychoanalysis

It is still difficult to question analysis in certain quarters. Once a therapist is committed to psychoanalysis, it is hard to turn back. For psychiatrists who have undergone formal training at an institute, questioning its principles and practice is almost impossible. On a purely emotional level, they have spent at least five years on a couch in personal treatment. To reject psychoanalysis would be to reject one's own training analyst who has spent years caring for one's psychological needs. (This is equally problematical for psychiatrists who have not gone to institutes, but have undergone personal analysis.) Moreover, trained analysts have lived for years in a culture where their professional peers and social networks have continuously reinforced a belief system. Those who reject it must leave the community and are condemned to be apostates.

Psychoanalysis is not quite finished in academic psychiatry. It is still a cohesive force in many departments, and analysts remain prominent as teachers. Still, its influence is becoming weaker as each new generation of practitioners and teachers comes of age. The change could take decades, but is probably inevitable. As a model of the mind, analysis is not consistent with cognitive theories or with the neurosciences. As a method of treating patients, it is elitist and of uncertain effectiveness. Thus, a renaissance seems unlikely.

What then has psychoanalysis bequeathed to psychiatry? Is it nothing but a set of ideas and methods that have become out of date? For the most part, yes. But psychoanalysis still has a legacy for psychiatry, and it should not be lost.

In chapter 5 I discussed the critique of contemporary psychiatry presented by the anthropologist Tania Luhrmann.[70] While I do not agree with Luhrmann that we should go back to teaching psychoanalysis, she is right to question whether psychiatrists are being properly trained. Even if formal psychotherapy is being given over to psychologists and other professionals, psychiatrists need a level of empathy that allows them to enter the inner world of patients.

Historically, psychoanalysis played a useful role in bringing psychotherapy into psychiatry. Without analysts, the field might well have developed in a purely biological direction, concentrating on hospitalized patients who need pharmacotherapy. As a psychiatrist who treats patients who require talking therapy as well as medication, I continue to make use of many skills I learned from my analytic teachers. It was from them that I learned to 'connect' with patients, by expressing interest non-verbally and by using words that reflect their inner world. To give psychoanalysts fair credit, they were pioneers in understanding subjective experiences, creating a tradition of approaching symptomatic patients as troubled people.

The caveat is that psychoanalysts have no patent on empathy. Non-analytic therapists, from the American Carl Rogers[71] to the Canadian Leslie Greenberg,[72] have placed empathy at the centre of theory and practice. Researchers in psychotherapy have shown that empathy is a crucial element that makes psychotherapy work.[73] There is also a tradition of 'phenomenology' in European psychiatry, begun by the German psychiatrist Karl Jaspers,[74] in which the patient's inner experience is placed at the centre of clinical interest.

The real problem with contemporary psychiatry is not that the field has lost its roots in psychoanalysis. It is that psychiatrists need to remember how to talk with their patients.

chapter 8

The State of Contemporary Psychiatry

The Place of Psychiatry in Medicine

Like many people who went into psychiatry in the 1960s, I was actually *happy* to enter a specialty that kept its distance from medicine. My experience as a student and as an intern in a teaching hospital showed me that doctors have little time to establish relationships with patients. We were too busy making sure that their body fluids were in balance to talk to them. Psychiatry, on the other hand, was about *life*.

It was only after many years in practice that I came to appreciate the value of the medical model. While talking to people is important, doing so hardly ever cures serious mental illness. Moreover, psychiatrists do not have unique insight into the human soul. That belief led our discipline astray, in a vain attempt to try to conquer the world.

By the end of the twentieth century psychiatry had returned to its natural place within medicine. In 1992, Sam Guze of Washington University published a book entitled *Why Psychiatry Is a Branch of Medicine.*[1] It would be difficult to imagine a similar book about why neurology or pediatrics belongs in medicine. When psychiatry identified with analysis, it was estranged from the medical family. Guze explained that it needed to come home.

Medicine generally understands disease as the result of disordered biochemistry and physiology. Yet a medical model does not exclude the role of psychological and social factors in illness. Life experiences bring on biological changes. In one study, normal subjects were asked to think depressing thoughts while undergoing PET scans – and the results of the imaging were much the same as in patients with clinical depression.[2] Thus, medicine does not need to split mind and body. By 1993, when I read an article by Guze entitled 'Biological Psychiatry: Is There Any Other Kind?'[3] my reaction was 'Right on!'

Not all my colleagues felt the same way. Opposition to the medical model in psychiatry came from two major constituencies: analysts and other therapists who attack the medical model as soulless and do not believe the mind can ever be understood as a product of the brain, as well as social psychiatrists who criticize the 'biomedical model' as dehumanizing and find psychiatry ignoring the social context of illness.

I have already examined the attempt of George Engel to develop a 'biopsychosocial' model of psychiatry to bridge these gaps and to be open to multiple perspectives.[4] What Engel failed to see is that biology takes priority in understanding mental illness,[5] because it explains why some people get sick under stressful life circumstances and others do not. The 'stress-diathesis' model of mental disorders[6] parallels most theories of illness in medicine – it explains the origin of illness on the basis of innate vulnerabilities that determine the type of disorder that could develop, and of environmental stressors that determine whether a disorder actually does develop.

Contemporary psychiatry is more respected and more secure within medicine than it was during the heyday of psychoanalysis. Yet psychiatry still occupies a relatively small niche. When there was only one way to become a doctor who cared about the mind and the soul, many humanistic medical students trained to be psychiatrists. Now there is an alternative, in family medicine. Thus, fewer medical graduates enter psychiatry.[7]

Psychiatry also continues to suffer from the stigma and fear associated with mental illness. Surveys shows that half the population will suffer from a diagnosable mental problem during a lifetime, and that at least 20 per cent will have a condition serious enough to require medical treatment.[8] One might expect a discipline that treats problems affecting so many people to be more attractive.

The problem is that medical students still see psychiatry as insufficiently scientific. We do not have an array of lab findings and physiological measurement to get young people excited. Moreover, faculty in other disciplines reinforce this perception. Any medical student who decides to go into the field must face a wall of opposition from teachers and colleagues. My most talented residents have told me that teachers have said, 'You're too smart to go into psychiatry.' Medical students who do choose psychiatry have to make a difficult transition between medicine and the less measurable world of the human mind.

Even today, physicians tend to equate psychiatry with psychoanalysis. For older faculty, trained in the 1960s and 1970s, this perception, however antiquated, conforms with their medical-school experiences. One prominent educator in my faculty told me that psychiatric residents are learning a lot of nonsense, and should spend more time working on medical wards. At the same time, psychoanalysts remain active and visible in the teaching of medical students. This does not go unnoticed by their medical colleagues. Fortunately, analytic ideas are not nearly as outrageous as they were in the past. (When I was a medical student, I was seriously informed that an X-ray picture of a peptic ulcer resembled a breast with a nipple, a resemblance that somehow explained why the ulcer developed in the first place.)

Where Is Psychiatry Going?

There was no such thing as psychiatry until the early 1900s.[9] About one hundred years earlier, at the end of the eighteenth century, a specialized corps of physicians in psychiatric hospitals had begun a new field; even so, psychiatry and neurology remained one discipline for many years.

Contemporary psychiatry stands on a boundary between the neurosciences and the social sciences. This is precisely what makes it exciting. Yet as we come to understand the mechanisms behind psychopathology, the domain of *mind* is shrinking and that of *brain* is expanding. Biology has emerged a clear winner in the struggle for the souls of psychiatrists.

To explain where psychiatry is going, I will examine four current trends: (1) links with the neurosciences; (2) the rise of evidence-based practice; (3) the increasing use of psychopharmacology; and (4) the changing role of psychotherapy.

Psychiatry and the Neurosciences

Academic psychiatrists were pleased when the first President Bush declared the 1990s 'The decade of the brain.'[10] Psychiatry had already turned back to biology, redefining itself as a discipline offering clinical applications of knowledge from the brain sciences. A neurologist colleague recently applauded my discipline with the suggestion: 'We take care of the neuron, and you look after the synapse.' (The synapse, or junction between nerve cells, is where many important psychiatric drugs are thought to have their effect.)

One only has to look at the covers of the *American Journal of Psychiatry* (now edited by a researcher in brain imaging) to see the change in psychiatrists' self-image. For some, their key icon was once a portrait of Sigmund Freud. (Henry Kravitz had a large bust in his office.) Today's icon, reflecting the new developments in psychiatry, is more likely to be dramatic colour pictures drawn from Positive Emission Tomography (PET) scans and Magnetic Resonance Imaging (MRI).

As an 'official' publication, the *Journal* still feels some responsibility to recognize psychoanalysis as a constituency (and to keep medical analysts as members of the American Psychiatric Association). While marginalizing psychoanalysis, the *Journal* only leaves space for it in the book-review section, and occasional two-page clinical conferences.

The same process has shaped academic psychiatry. University departments are no longer enclaves for introspection, but centres for basic research on the brain. As we learn to read the genome, psychiatrists are beginning to understand mental illness in a new way.[11] Diagnosis and classification will come to reflect genetic differences linked to characteristic patterns on brain scans. Treatment will be guided by data from genetics and imaging. At this point, most of this research is decades away from having any meaningful clinical application. Yet my own department recently considered recruiting a PhD chemist whose research uses viruses as 'vectors' to carry new genes into the brain. We could be treating patients with schizophrenia and bipolar illness with gene therapy in the foreseeable future.

When I was an undergraduate student in psychology in the late 1950s, it seemed obvious that the patients at Ypsilanti State Hospital had defective brains. But it has taken many decades for science to come up with any sort of explanation as to what is wrong. And we still don't really know. The complexity of the defects in mental illness is mind-boggling. Not only is very little still known about how different parts of the brain function, but every region is linked to every other: it has been estimated that the number of connections between the billions of neurons in the human brain is greater than the number of stars in the universe.[12]

In the 1950s and 1960s, brain research took a new direction into chemistry. The discovery that drugs could control schizophrenia was at first no more than an unexplained, albeit fortunate, observation. Little had been known about how neurons connected with each other at the synapse. It had once been thought that nerve impulses jump the gap as electrical sparks. Then, as it became clear that chemicals were usually needed to make these connections, the functioning of neurotransmitters became a central issue for psychiatry.

Science advances most when it works with an attractive theory. In the 1960s and 1970s, the idea became current that depression is due to defects in noradrenaline and/or serotonin, and that schizophrenia resulted from defects in dopamine transmission.[13] These proposals were based on the actions of drugs (it was thought that antidepressants increase the release of noradrenaline and serotonin, while antipsychotics block dopamine.) While these theories ultimately proved too simple, they made neuroscience and psychopharmacology into major areas of research.

Many prominent leaders in academic psychiatry are experts in neurochemistry and on the relationship between defects in synaptic transmission and major mental disorders. These subjects have become progressively more complicated, and any serious researcher needs to be highly focused. For this reason, there are chairs of psychiatry in the United States who know more about ions than about people. When one of them stepped down recently, I heard his colleagues say, 'Poor guy, now he has to see patients again.' In a more troubling development, some universities have considered hiring PhD researchers, who have never seen a patient or made a diagnosis, to head departments of psychiatry.

The neurosciences are driving the agenda of psychiatric research. The hot topics are genetics and imaging. The human genome has been read, and it is known that about half of our genes are involved in brain function.[14] In the coming years, their precise function will be understood, and the new discipline of 'Proteiomics' will discover the functions of the proteins that these genes construct.[15] PET and MRI scans can already trace the pathways of transmitters and drugs. Psychiatry is well on the way to explaining madness through molecules.

The prestige of biological psychiatry has been built on these advances. The success of 'designer drugs' such as Prozac is linked in most clinician's minds to brain science.[16] Many of the drugs psychiatrists use treat diseases that talking therapy doesn't even touch.

While our discipline is less crazy than it used to be, it isn't always as much fun. I still love to teach on patients, a situation where I am allowed to speculate about what makes people tick. I may have done too much of this, given how far I had fallen behind on the latest developments. Like most of my colleagues, I kept up with biological psychiatry, at least to the extent of learning how to prescribe the latest drugs. (I was frankly amazed at the results I obtained by prescribing Prozac and its relatives.) Yet I did not realize how fast brain science was moving. The most common chemical transmitter in the human brain was almost unknown until ten years ago.[17] And it has recently been discovered that, contrary to everything we were taught, new brain cells can grow in adult life.[18]

Is this a good-news story? Yes and no. There has also been criticism of the way psychiatry is going, not all of which has come from psychoanalysts.

Not all aspects of human behaviour can be explained by molecules. *Reductionist* science assumes that complex phenomena can be understood by reducing them to simple mechanisms.[19] This is not always a bad thing. Chemistry was one of the great triumphs of reductionism: reactions that once had seemed mysterious and magical were explained by the periodic table of elements and by the structure of molecules.

Medicine as a whole has gone mad over molecules. But mental illness is different. Even as a student, I could not see how studying the movement of ions across the membranes of neurons could explain the complexities of human behaviour. There are many aspects of psychiatry that require research at the level of the individual, or even the social community. At these levels, systems have 'emergent properties.'[20] Simply put, the whole is greater than the sum of its parts.

I have had trouble defending our approach to colleagues from other medical disciplines. I was recently chatting with the director of a research institute who is an expert on AIDS. He could not understand why all questions about mental disorders cannot be studied using molecular methods. He was truly puzzled as to how research on psychotherapy, or on culture and psychiatry, could possibly be useful. My colleague is not alone in his confusion. What he failed to understand was the difference between applying the principles of scientific research to psychiatry and coming up with strictly biological explanations for behaviour.

Psychiatry may be going molecular, but it also needs to keep in touch with the social sciences. There is no theoretical difficulty in explaining the function of the liver or the kidney at a cellular or molecular level. To do the same for the human brain and for thought and emotions is another matter. That is where psychology comes in. Biological research runs the risk of leaving little room for the study of people, not to speak of the human condition – the issue at the core of psychoanalysis.

As psychiatrists develop more powerful tools to change behaviour, they are becoming more like their medical colleagues. There was a time when we were the only ones who talked to patients (even if we could not do much else for them). Today, I often hear patients complaining about psychiatrists who see them for fifteen minutes and write a prescription to get them out of the office.

Psychiatry has long had an identity problem. It has always been a 'boundary discipline,' linking biology, psychology, and culture. If it were to abdicate this role, it might as well pack its bags and give the whole enterprise back to neurology.

Evidence-Based Practice

In the last thirty years, no medical specialty has changed as much as psychiatry. While internists and pediatricians have much greater knowledge than they once did, they are still working within the same paradigm. But psychiatrists of the previous generation have had to move from practice rooted in intuition to practice based on evidence. They are like time travellers who find themselves in an almost unrecognizable world.

With the rise of evidence-based medicine, all physicians are expected to conform to standards based on evidence and to be accountable for the outcome if they do not. Psychiatrists face precisely the same challenge.[21]

The Osheroff case (see chapter 5) dramatized this issue. The psychiatrists treating Osheroff should have prescribed antidepressants because research had established their efficacy for the melancholic depression from which he suffered. The physicians in charge of the case failed to make the right diagnosis, and provided ineffective therapy that led to unnecessary suffering. It was not really defensible for Alan Stone to describe their practice as the view of a 'respectable minority.'[22]

As we collect more data, psychiatrists will have to restrict their options and practice in accordance with what research tells them is effective. When I was a resident, it was not unusual for psychoanalysts to tell prospective patients that they would not improve unless they came several times a week for full analytic treatment. This opinion was never based on evidence of any kind, but followed from a strong ideological position. Analysts truly believed their method was life-saving. As one of them said to me, 'How can you talk about symptoms, when a person's whole life is at stake?' Analysts also felt that they should offer their patients nothing less than the same treatment that they themselves received as part of their training. Even then, however, not everyone wanted to be analysed. Outside of a core constituency of analytic groupies, patients offered a recommendation of frequent sessions over several years would ask, 'Am I really that sick?' For the analysts, questions like this only proved how afraid patients were to explore their unconscious.

A psychoanalyst who practised like that today might well face a lawsuit. This possibility is well known in the analytic community. Analysts who have kept up with psychiatry often prescribe medication in combination with talking therapy. Others, believing that giving drugs spoils the purity of the analytic relationship, will refer their patient to a colleague who provides the necessary prescription. Moreover, as the number of non-physicians who train as analysts becomes a majority, 'split treatments' are becoming more and more frequent.[23]

Psychiatrists, like other physicians, are now practising in a much less authoritarian fashion. Patients rightly expect to be provided with information about options and to make choices. It will not be unusual in the future for psychiatrist and patient to sit in front of a computer screen and review data relevant to a decision. (One of my former students, now a leading psychiatrist in Toronto, already practises in this way.) This is a far cry from the way medicine used to be practised, in that physicians were simply trusted on the basis of their expert knowledge.

Psychoanalysis corresponded to this older authoritarian model. The patient lay passively on a couch, while the analyst, out of sight, took notes, listened, and eventually commented. Interpretations were provided *ex cathedra*, and, given the analyst's long period of training, had to be correct. When patients had different opinions, they were assumed to be 'resisting.'

Traditionally, patients have been at the mercy of the physician's knowledge (or lack of knowledge). Few practitioners of medicine outside academia are great readers of journal articles. Many depend on free updates provided in the mail, or even on information from pharmaceutical representatives. But patients are now empowered by the Internet. Many come to physicians armed with information they have gleaned there. In this new climate, physicians either have to keep up or look ignorant.

Unfortunately, what patients find on the Net is not always that accurate. There are reputable sites with state-of-the-art information,[24] and there are also chat lines where people trade opinions and personal stories. In my own area of interest, borderline personality disorder, I encourage patients to look up their diagnosis on line. Most are surprised and relieved to find there are really other people with the same problems. But I have also had patients who have found false and misleading information on the Net.

Computers and the Internet have affected almost everything in the modern world, and psychiatry is no exception. The algorithims for diagnosis in DSM function as analogues of computer science. In coming

decades, computerized diagnoses may replace the still unreliable judgment of clinical observers. Computers are also likely to affect clinical
decisions. As the practice of psychiatry becomes more evidence-based,
practitioners will come to depend on data available on-line.

All the same, physicians will always rely on clinical judgment. After
years of experience, one can make a diagnosis five minutes into an interview, and usually get it right. This comes from seeing myriad cases that
eventually fall into patterns. Similarly, experienced physicians usually
know what treatment to offer a patient, even if they have to stop and
think about how they reached their conclusions.

Evidence-based medicine still has a long way to go. Controlled trials
of treatment are complex and expensive. We lack good ones for most of
the drugs and therapies physicians offer. Moreover, treatments that
work under rigidly controlled conditions with carefully selected patients
may turn out to be unhelpful in the hurly-burly of practice, where
patients are usually much sicker than the ones who sign up for clinical
trials.

Nonetheless, psychiatry is becoming more and more evidence-based.
And the process is only beginning. The change is already reflected in
the textbooks we use, and the journals we read. The process is the same
everywhere. Textbooks of psychiatry today have little clinical opinion,
and a mountain of facts. The evolution of the *American Journal of Psychiatry* (described in chapter 1) has been paralleled by similar developments
at the *British Journal* and at the *Canadian Journal.* Opinion pieces and
clinical vignettes have disappeared, replaced by methodological rigour,
quantitative data, and conclusions open to revision by further research.
Psychiatry is now in the mainstream of medicine and science.

Psychopharmacology and Psychiatry

People once stereotyped psychiatrists as thoughtful men sitting behind
couches. Now half of us are women, and we talk to our patients face to
face. Moreover, the popular image of psychiatry centres around the prescription of drugs. Whereas the mystique of the psychiatrist once
derived from unique insight into the workings of the mind, it now
depends on the power of medication.

Over the course of my career as a psychiatrist, I have lived through the
great developments in psychopharmacology. I am old enough to have
seen schizophrenics unmedicated and desperate in a state hospital.
Then, as a medical student, I saw the early miracles of antipsychotic

treatment, when the treatment of psychosis became a matter of weeks rather than of months or years. As a resident, I was the first person at my hospital to prescribe lithium for a patient with bipolar disorder.

Yet every good idea in psychiatry has a bad side. In the 1940s we knew that electro-convulsive therapy (ECT) pulls people out of severe depression. Used properly, ECT remains one of the most effective treatments in psychiatry.[25] But before antidepressants were introduced, any patient who was depressed might be given ECT. A similar problem has occurred with lithium. It is so effective in bipolar illness that some psychiatrists seem to want to diagnose everyone with the disorder, just so they can give them lithium (or other mood stabilizers such as valproate). The result has been that people who don't need these drugs end up taking them.

We still see patients who refuse to take any drug that might affect their mind, believing that their autonomy is at stake. By and large, however, the public has embraced psychopharmacology. Whereas cocktail-party chatter among patients might have once centred on the progress of their analysis, one might now hear discussions of the relative merits of various antidepressants.

There is nothing intrinsically wrong with psychopharmacology. Anyone who starts the morning with a cup of coffee is already applying it to their own lives. The question is whether the aura of scientific precision that accompanies contemporary practice is justified.

Psychiatrists have an armamentarium of agents that would have astonished the practitioners of fifty years ago. Antipsychotic drugs were a tremendous breakthrough – they may not cure schizophrenia, but they keep patients out of hospital. The same can be said for lithium and bipolar disorder. The antidepressants of today are probably not superior to what we used forty years ago, but their reduced side effects mean that patients are more likely to take them rather than throw them away.

Drugs are useful, but the companies that make them give out a terrible amount of hype. Moreover, the physicians who prescribe them expect too much. Sometimes pharmacological treatment achieves a cure. More often it takes the edge off mental pain without removing it. And sometimes it accomplishes nothing at all.

The most commonly prescribed drugs are antidepressants. Used properly, these are marvellous agents. They should really be called 'antineurotics,' since they are also effective against anxiety, phobias, and obsessive-compulsive symptoms, and even help to stop bulimics from binging.[26] Yet antidepressants do not always work. Complete recoveries

occur only about half the time, with many patients remaining symptomatic, even on adequate doses.[27] In general, antidepressants are better for
depressions with a recent onset, and not so effective for chronic symptoms.[28] Psychiatrists are sometimes taught to handle 'treatment resistance' by either increasing doses or giving two, three, or four drugs
when one doesn't do the trick. This 'algorithmic' approach does not
always work.[29] But patients, and their psychiatrists, keep on trying. Many
have their drugs adjusted on every visit yet never really get better. (This
is one of the reasons I got interested in personality disorders, a concept
that helps explain why some patients do not respond to pharmacological treatment.)

We still do not know enough about what causes mental illness. Psychiatrists may be repeating the mistakes of the past by being as arrogant
about their drugs as they once were about their talking therapies. That
said, psychopharmacology is, by and large, a success story. Drugs do not
cure diseases, but they certainly reduce distress. The irony is that we still
know little about how they work. The oldest biological treatment in psychiatry is ECT, and we still don't have a clue how it brings people out of
depression.

Paradoxically, I find this picture comforting. If we can do *this* well
without understanding how drugs work, how much better will we do
when the mysteries of the brain begin to be unravelled? The limitations
of psychopharmacology are growing pains. In time, we psychiatrists will
have more sophisticated and more effective options.

A Changing Role for Psychotherapy

Psychotherapy has become a crowded marketplace. Psychoanalysis has
been undermined by competition from other therapies, some of which
have a stronger evidence base for their effectiveness. Analysis will not
find its way back into the mainstream of psychiatry without strong data
to prove that it works.

Psychotherapy is an art, but must also be a science. The research literature in the field is almost as large as that for psychopharmacology.
Most of this work has been done by psychologists, often outside of medical schools. The psychotherapy research community is no longer very
interested in analytic therapy. Whereas the standard text (*Handbook of
Psychotherapy and Behavior Change*) used to have a chapter on research in
psychoanalytic therapy, the fifth edition, published in 2003, barely men-
tions the subject.[30]

Cognitive behavioural therapy has stimulated the largest amount of research. CBT started as a treatment for depression, and then became a general therapy for many conditions.[31] It takes relatively little interest in the quality of a patient's childhood or the way people relate to their therapists. The emphasis is on the here-and-now. Depressed patients receiving CBT will be asked to re-examine they way they think about their current life and themselves, and will be actively encouraged to develop new problem-solving strategies. CBT patients do not lie on a couch, but are given instructions and homework.

When I was a resident, we had behaviour therapy, which was based on the ideas of a Russian physiologist (Ivan Pavlov) and a Harvard psychology professor (B.F. Skinner). But behaviour therapy was only interested in behaviour, that is, stimulus, response, and reinforcement.[32] It treated the brain as a 'black box' that could be safely ignored. The behavioural psychologist I described in chapter 5 could not believe that patients actually heard voices. (Evidently, belief in absurd ideas is not limited to psychoanalysts.) Aaron Beck's cognitive therapy corrected this error by placing the mind at the centre of theory and practice.

I have never been formally trained in CBT, but I have learned to incorporate its principles into my work with patients. When a patient with borderline personality cuts her wrists, you won't get very far by talking about whether she is angry at you or her mother. Instead, you need to go back over the emotional state that led up to the cutting, and explore with patients how they might have dealt with it differently.[33]

When I read books about CBT, I discovered that I was already doing many of the things they were suggesting. Like many therapists, I became more practical over time, spending less time talking about the past and more focusing on solving problems in the present, and I challenged the way patients thought about themselves and the world around them.

Historically, behavioural and cognitive therapies have been the province of psychologists, defining a separate identity for clinical psychology. Beck's students, and most of the current leaders in the field, have been psychologists. But psychiatrists, impressed with the strong evidence for the effectiveness of CBT, have come to use it too. Residents demand training in the method, and psychiatry departments have hired cognitive psychologists to teach CBT. The traditional practice of teaching psychiatric residents analytic therapy only is dying out. The main exception in Canada is McGill, almost the only department in Canada that continues to devote a large amount of attention to psychoanalysis. (We attract residents from other provinces who cannot find analytic teaching elsewhere.)

The profusion of psychotherapies has reflected an overall failure of the field to be guided by research. If therapists conducted an evidence-based practice, there would be a very short list of options for them to follow. Faddism remains a problem. In the 1990s a few psychiatrists advocated spending years hypnotizing patients to help them to 'recover' memories of child abuse.[34] Often combined with techniques that encouraged patients to develop multiple personalities, the recovered-memory movement created one of the great scandals in the history of psychotherapy.[35] And as Frederick Crews pointed out, its basic ideas came directly from Freud.[36]

New therapy fads continue to appear. One of the newer methods, Francine Shapiro's EMDR (Eye Movement Desensitization and Reprocessing),[37] has therapists waving a wand in front of patients who are supposed to be reliving traumatic experiences. Research has shown that this method, while it has some therapeutic value, is no better than other standard approaches, and that eye movements have nothing to do with its effectiveness.[38] One wonders if EMDR is little more than a recreation of the suggestive methods used before the French Revolution by the famous Austrian hypnotist Anton Mesmer.[39]

Fortunately, most psychotherapy researchers are commendably hard-headed. Marsha Linehan, a cognitive therapist from Seattle who has used a form of CBT for borderline personality disorder,[40] has conducted randomized controlled trials supported by the NIMH, publishing her results in the *Archives of General Psychatry* and *the American Journal of Psychiatry*. Linehan, who speaks all over the country, is often asked by members of her audience to respond to approaches different from her own. Her response is, 'That's a good idea, and I hope you do research about it, just as I have.'

Linehan believes that in the future there will be only one type of psychotherapy for any condition in psychiatry, and its effectiveness will be shown through research data.[41] She is appalled by the fact that patients can receive entirely contradictory recommendations from different therapists. This problem still affects medicine (not all doctors can be counted on to come up with the same answer), but evidence-based practice is gradually making the situation better for patients.

Psychopharmacology in Contemporary Practice

Biological treatments may be more effective than psychoanalysis, but they do not always work. Unfortunately, psychiatrists don't always seem to know the limitations of drugs, and keep on prescribing them. This is part of a larger problem. Most physicians do not consistently practise evidence-based medicine. To follow those principles, they would have to tolerate doubt and be much more conservative in practice.

As Robert Michels notes,[42] most doctors do not really follow scientific developments, but are satisfied to know what experts think. And their patients do not easily allow them to be conservative. People suffering from symptoms come in wanting the 'right' drug, and if they don't get it, they seek treatment elsewhere.

Drug companies have had a tremendous influence on medical practice. Their advertisements, and even more so the use of 'detail men' to market their products directly to physicians, have been shown to be highly effective.[43] Moreover, the industry is constantly looking for new marketing niches for their products, such as drugs for social anxiety.[44]

Academic psychiatry cannot afford to ignore the pharmaceutical industry. It is no longer possible to run a large medical conference without large amounts of support from these companies. Moreover, the industry is now allowed to pitch directly to the consumer through advertising. (We do not permit these ads in Canada, but our patients watch American TV and read American magazines.) Ultimately the problem is that non-pharmacological therapies require people to administer them, and people cost money. Prescribing a drug often seems like the cheapest alternative.

The result is that patients with mental disorders are receiving too many drugs. They also are not getting enough psychotherapy, even the types that have been shown to be effective. In my own area of borderline personality disorder, chronically suicidal patients are being prescribed four or five drugs,[45] none of which really works very well.[46] And no one spends much time talking to these patients, unless they come in to the emergency room threatening to kill themselves (which is exactly what some do).

In this context, a residual nostalgia for psychoanalysis begins to make sense.[47] Analysts are interested in people and know how to talk to them. That is why residents still value them as teachers. The problem is that psychiatry has gone from one extreme to another. One can only hope that, with time, the situation will get back into balance.

The Psychiatry of the Future

When I trained as a resident, I expected to devote most of my career to psychotherapy. I wanted to see patients who were deeply troubled but functional. Today's residents expect to be experts in psychopharmacology, as well as leaders of teams in hospitals and clinics. Most of their patients will be either psychotic or severely depressed. Few young psychiatrists think of opening up an outside office to conduct psychotherapy. The small number who still train as analysts have no expectation of developing a full-time practice. Young psychiatrists are facing a different world.

Patients seeking help for mental problems are also facing a different environment. They are unlikely to meet a psychoanalyst who will recommend years of treatment for relatively minor problems. Some patients may never even see a psychiatrist unless their difficulties are severe. Psychiatrists are spending more and more of their time on illnesses like schizophrenia and bipolar disorder. Most people with depression are being seen by family doctors or non-medical professionals, and may only run into a psychiatrist if they need a consultation.

Psychiatrists have also been moving away from psychotherapy. In the United States, managed care has made sure of that, by instituting restrictions on how long patients can be seen.[48] (Although insurance for extended therapy should not be routine, insuring less than ten sessions goes against what scientific evidence shows about psychological interventions.)[49] In Canada, since their numbers are relatively small, few patients can actually obtain access to free therapy. Thus, in both countries, most people receiving psychotherapy have to seek treatment from psychologists and social workers.

How will this scenario change in the coming decades? Treacherous as it is to predict the future, three current trends seem likely to continue. First, psychiatric practice will become more evidence-based. Second, treatments will be based on neuroscience. Third, psychiatrists will concentrate on the sickest patients.

The last point is crucial. Psychiatrists have been attacked for concentrating on the 'worried well' and abandoning the mentally ill.[50] Psychoanalysis is a treatment for high-functioning patients. As long as this was the model, psychiatrists were unlikely to fulfil their responsibility to the severely ill. Most other physicians have always believed that the sickest cases deserved the highest priority.

As psychiatrists become experts in severe mental illness, they function less as direct caregivers and more as consultants. In the past, psychiatry has been a 'first-line' specialty, that is, patients came directly for help without being referred. That situation is changing. More and more patients are sent by family doctors when first-line treatments fail. We are also asked to step in to help psychologists and social workers who run into trouble with patients in psychotherapy.

It follows that psychiatry may not need so many practitioners in order to care for the mentally ill. In the future, they will carry fewer patients, treating only those who require their specialized knowledge and skills. Care needs to be delegated and apportioned to other professionals. This means getting out of private offices and working in teams at hospitals or clinics.

Organized psychiatry is making a big mistake by fighting other disciplines for market share. As Heinz Lehmann realized twenty years ago, psychiatrists will always be expensive and scarce.[51] Therefore, their precious time has to be assigned to tasks that others cannot do, most particularly emergency treatment and management of the most severely ill patients. In a time when family doctors comfortably prescribe antidepressants, and when psychologists are at least as competent in psychotherapy, psychiatry should be working out a unique niche for itself.

In Canada, psychiatrists are not looking for work – they already have too much to do. In the United States, however, they are both underinsured and facing competition from clinical psychologists and social workers. It is interesting that ever since September 11, 2001, the American Psychiatric Association has been trumpeting a need for psychiatrists in America to deal with the effects of trauma. Virtually every issue of *Psychiatric News*, the newsletter provided to all APA members, has picked up on this theme.[52] One gets the impression that disasters are good for business. Yet there is really no reason why traumatized people need to see psychiatrists, or why they need them more than other professionals. Psychiatrists have been leaders in research on trauma, but they are no better than anyone else at managing it. Moreover, a large percentage of people exposed to trauma avoid therapists, and may even do better by *not* dwelling on negative experiences.[53] Time may not heal all wounds, but it usually makes them less raw.

Psychiatrists in the future will need to concentrate on their unique mission. No other group of physicians or therapists knows as much as we do about the treatment of severe mental illness. I expect that we will return even more strongly to our medical roots, and help other disciplines to manage patients with less-severe illnesses. Breakthroughs in understanding the brain could be as decisive as the discovery of DNA. In 2050, the psychiatry of 2000 will appear as backward to psychiatrists of the day as the theory and practice of 1950 seem to us now. Psychoanalysts have sometimes talked about the publication of Freud's *Interpreta-*

tion of Dreams in 1900 as an event that inaugurated a new century. But we find ourselves in still another century. The psychoanalytic era has past, and a new one has begun. And in light of what we know today, Freud heralded a false dawn.

Afterword: Why They Believed

The God That Failed

A book entitled *The God That Failed*,[1] published a few years after the end of the Second World War, presented a series of essays by prominent intellectuals who had at first embraced, and then rejected, communism. No such book has yet appeared about psychoanalysis. Yet its decline parallels that other great disillusionment of modern times. Psychoanalysis and socialism both lie outside the boundaries of science. They are belief systems that attempt to cope with a loss of faith and to give meaning to the human condition.

As the analytic movement, like socialism, lost its cultural hegemony, even those who had been strongly attracted to it became opponents. My own experiences were typical of my generation. I graduated from medical school in the 1960s, at a time when young people took it for granted that the world was about to be transformed. If society or the economy created injustice and poverty, people of good will would fight to make things right. If you were in personal trouble, you could seek therapy or psychoanalysis.

Still, I was brought up to be a sceptic. I worked with analysts and admired many of them, but could never have tolerated training in an institute. I kept my distance, trying to find my own truth and my own version of therapy. All the same, the social climate kept me in the role of a supporter. It took me years to break away from psychoanalysis, and doing so was painful. I regret not seeing through my illusions sooner, but I was a child of my time. I could only make the paradigm shift when psychiatry changed around me.

The Decline of Religion

The decline of organized religion in the Western world has been a gradual process, and it is not yet over.[2] The Reformation had challenged the dominance of the single faith of Roman Catholicism. In the eighteenth century, Enlightenment intellectuals such as Voltaire, Rousseau, and Diderot also attacked the Catholic church, but these men were Deists, not atheists. They did not question the existence of God, but the role of organized religion as an obstacle to the advancement of human knowledge.

By the mid-nineteenth century, leading intellectuals could be frank unbelievers. Charles Darwin, the most influential thinker of his time, rejected religious belief after the death of a favourite daughter.[3] The Victorian writer Matthew Arnold (1822–88), in his famous poem 'Dover Beach,'[4] pictured the fading of faith as a vast receding ebb-tide, leaving humanity desolate on the shore:

> The Sea of Faith
> was once, too, at the full, and round earth's shore
> Lay like the folds of a bright girdle furl'd.
> But now I only hear
> Its melancholy, long, withdrawing roar,
> Retreating, to the breath
> Of the night-wind, down the vast edges drear
> And naked shingles of the world.

Arnold believed that the only comfort for the loss of religion would have to come from personal attachments:

> Ah, love, let us be true
> To one another! for the world, which seems
> To lie before us like a land of dreams,
> So various, so beautiful, so new,
> Hath really neither joy, nor love, nor light,
> Nor certitude, nor peace, nor help for pain;
> And we are here as on a darkling plain
> Swept with confused alarms of struggle and flight,
> Where ignorant armies clash by night.

Ironically, as sociologists have observed,[5] Arnold's solution does not quite work. As the social cohesion of Western society has decreased, people have come to depend more on personal rather than on social supports. This trend has created an intolerable burden for marriage and the family, making their dissolution more likely.

By the end of the nineteenth century, Nietzsche had declared the 'death of God,'[6] and the arts reflected a vast spiritual crisis. Then, in the first decades of the twentieth century, a movement known as *modernism*[7] swept away all the certainties of the past. In the world that modernity created, no belief and loyalty remained secure. As individualism has replaced collectivism, the impact of modernism creates world-wide and rapid social change, and challenges all traditional religions.

Most people still believe in God, and their faith provides them with comfort in times of trouble; religious belief has been shown to be strongly protective against mental illness.[8] Membership in religious movements also provides a social glue and sense of belonging. Yet the frequency and intensity of formal affiliation to organized religion has changed. Church attendance has dramatically fallen in most European countries, and in most parts of the Western Hemisphere (the United States being the great exception).[9] Religious fundamentalism may only be a rearguard action against the relentless advance of modernity. Yet the loss of organized religion left behind an enormous gap. New ideologies were needed to fill this vacuum.

Marxism was one such belief.[10] It emerged at the same time as the decline of faith and then, for a time, commanded the allegiance of a large portion of humanity. Marx's ideas were presented as science, but constituted a secular religion marked by sacred texts, popes, and schisms. Marxism was a political and economic system that espoused the belief in a perfect society that could only be realized through revolutionary change. Unlike traditional religion, the Marxist faith did not rationalize misfortune by expecting justice in the afterlife. In a world where God was absent, virtue would be rewarded in a utopian future. The concept of creating paradise in this world, instead of the next, offered a secular alternative to religion. Marx saw history as an eschatological drama in which the victory of the revolution would follow a final confrontation between the forces of good and evil. He was hostile to organized religion, which he saw as supportive of the status quo. Marxism has rarely attracted religious believers. Its adherents searched for a commitment to create meaning in a world shorn of faith and certainty.

How Psychoanalysis Became a Religion

Psychoanalysis appeared on the scene a few decades after Marxism, but the peak of its influence on Western culture occurred in the mid-twentieth century, contemporaneous with a further decline of religious belief. The analytic movement was an ideological force that offered a different form of perfectibility.[11] Instead of bringing about a social utopia, analysis became associated with the idea of psychological perfection, that is, of being 'completely analysed.' In an essay written in his twilight years, Martin Grotjahn,[12] a German émigré who made a career in California, lamented ironically that his impending death was a waste, given how well he had analysed himself over the years.

To be fair, this was not Freud's view: he had famously stated that he only wished to replace neurosis with normal human unhappiness.[13] But as psychoanalysis turned into a social movement, its ideas took on a utopian cast. The British anthropologist Ernest Gellner, a trenchant and witty critic of psychoanalysis, understood this problem.[14] Gellner argued that analytic therapy plays a particular role in modernist society by offering ways to manage anxiety, a function that is particularly important in the face of the increased complexity of human relationships in a society lacking clearcut rules. One might add that in a world without ultimate meaning, people could still strive to find personal happiness by being in control of their psyches.

Freud, Jewish but a non-believer, created a movement that provided the personal and spiritual guidance previously offered by religion. In the Catholic environment of Vienna, he created a new form of confession, with a listening analyst-priest sitting out of direct view. Yet psychoanalysis has always had a special appeal for Jewish people. Alienated from the mainstream of their societies, the European Jews were an intellectual and social avant-garde that anticipated important cultural developments. Most early psychoanalysts were non-believing Jewish intellectuals, uncomfortable with their own religious traditions, but attracted to other world views.

Even today, a disproportionately high percentage of analytic therapists and patients are Jewish.[15] I have heard analysts half-jokingly refer to their institutes as 'synagogues.' Among patients, the Woody Allen stereotype is only funny because it is half-true. Psychoanalysis has always appealed to people who are marginalized and alienated.

The non-Jewish members of the early psychoanalytic movement were also alienated from their religious traditions. Carl Gustav Jung, the son of a Protestant minister, was an early and prominent convert.[16] But the schismatic movement he later created had an overtly religious cast. Jung came to believe that analysis could actually bring people back to God.

Even scientifically trained psychiatrists are not entirely immune to this temptation. I recently attended a presentation by a professor of psychiatry who also happens to be a strong Christian. The presenter talked to his audience about the need to teach patients with personality disorders to restore contact with God and spirituality. It was a little surprising to see a researcher leading a large group of psychiatrists at an international meeting in meditation exercises.

Over time, Freud's movement took on more and more of the trappings of a religious sect. The first task of every analytic candidate is to read the master's works from cover to cover. My colleagues who studied at the institute had to absorb every word. Freud's voluminous writings also became the subject of endless commentary and exegesis by his followers, creating a literature that can only be described as Talmudic.

The process of analytic training, with its rituals and long period of personal sacrifice, parallels preparations for the priesthood. My colleagues who went through this process were expected to treat Freud with reverence. Frequent references to his published papers are codes signalling a deep sense of belonging.

Finally, and most tellingly, psychoanalysis underwent a series of schisms reminiscent of the Protestant Reformation and its aftermath. Heretics were no longer burned, but they could be excommunicated and shunned. After the death of Freud, psychoanalysts could propose radically new theories while remaining within the movement. By the 1970s, conducting an *auto-da-fé* of a dissident was unheard of, and it became possible to disagree with Freud and remain an analyst. But psychoanalysis, like Christianity, had long since splintered into hundreds of sub-sects, each form having its own brand name, and each claiming to have developed a unique method of therapy for the human condition.

Some analysts revised Freud, placing the most crucial problems of childhood during infancy. As the source of trouble was pushed further and further into an unremembered past, proof or disproof of any model became even less possible. Obviously, these ideas were still a form of psychoanalysis. While some might be described as 'kinder and gentler,' as opposed to the fierce and dark world view proposed by Freud, none of these revisions changed the quasi-religious nature of the psychoanalytic movement.

Any continuing attachment to organized religion tended to conflict with psychoanalysis. Jung's espousal of spirituality had led to the first major schism in the movement. These ideas live on, not only in the continued popularity of books inspired by Jungian ideas, but in 'New Age' psychology, and in the fusion of psychotherapy and spirituality advocated by psychiatrists such as M. Scott Peck.[17]

By and large, religious belief has been regarded by psychoanalysts as an area either to be analysed away or to be left alone. Only a few analysts have been strongly religious. An example in the McGill community was Karl Stern, a Holocaust survivor who converted to Catholicism during the Second World War and wrote a widely read autobiography about his experiences.[18] As late as 1970, Stern told a colleague from another converted family of German Jews that his treatment would be fine as long as the analyst was a Catholic. (My colleague ended up seeing a Protestant, after which, as Stern feared, he left the church.)

Some analysts added a political dimension to psychoanalysis. Alfred Adler, Karen Horney, and Erich Fromm[19] were socialists who believed that society, not just individuals, needed to change before most people could become mentally healthy. These ideas regained popularity in the 1960s when they were taken up by cultural gurus such as Herbert Marcuse, Norman Brown, and R.D. Laing.[20]

But two ideologies that step into the same breach are not necessarily compatible. Marxists who moved too close to psychoanalysis might be criticized by their socialist colleagues for being too concerned with their own psyches, as opposed to advocating the need for basic change in society. Analysts who became Marxists sometimes had to leave the movement. Erich Fromm, who espoused a humanistic interpretation of Marx, was forced to create his own splinter movement.[21] Wilhelm Reich flirted with communism, and then went on to create his own messianic new-age movement.[22] Most of the left-wing people I knew from the 1960s who went into analysis ended up concentrating on their own psyches to the exclusion of larger issues. In some cases, they eventually became distinctly right-wing.

The Triumph of Science

Scientific empiricism is a way of knowing that does not rely on scripture, revelation, or authority. One can hypothesize as creatively as one wishes, but data is the final arbiter of truth.

As its benefits to humanity have mounted, the position of science in modern society has become almost unchallengeable. Instead of rejecting science, ideologies try to appropriate it. Socialism and psychoanalysis both emerged at a time when science had already developed great prestige. Part of the appeal of Marx's ideas was the belief that 'scientific socialism' had discovered principles that could explain and even predict the course of world history. Freud, who had a scientific training, also claimed to have discovered an empirical method that could provide access to hidden corners of the mind, and explain present behaviour on the basis of past experience. The supposed therapeutic efficacy of Freud's method was also the basis of its claim to be scientific.

Marxism failed the test of empiricism when every attempt at implementing its ideas ended in failure. While true believers may claim that 'socialism has never really been tried,' history has shown that it has usually led to economic decline and despotism.

Psychoanalysis also failed to meet the test of empiricism, leading to its replacement by biological psychiatry. There have been problems with this shift, but many of them are due to oversimplifications of empirical ideas. Scientific psychiatry is not the same as the definitions of the DSM manual, a theory of the brain, or of a plan of drug treatment. Science is about testing hypotheses and changing them when new evidence comes in. You can do that on any level, from molecule to society.

I became a researcher after stumbling into science. Nothing in my residency, most of which took place in psychoanalytically oriented settings, prepared me for the idea that problems require systematic investigation. For the next ten years, I was happy to work as a therapist and a teacher. I also thought the workings of the mind were much too complex to be submitted to research. A psychologist I knew remarked wrly, 'The researchable questions aren't that important, and the important questions aren't that researchable.'

I changed my mind for two reasons. First, I discovered that science *can* address clinically important issues. Second, I became disillusioned with the results of psychoanalytic therapy, and realized that these deficiencies were not just a reflection of my own limitations. At mid-life I turned to science and to evidence-based psychiatry. Since then I have had the conviction of a convert.

In order to understand why some of my colleagues do not agree with me, I have thought about why they went into psychiatry. As a group, I have always found psychiatrists are more creative and interesting than other physicians. (I may be prejudiced on this subject.) Psychiatry attracts people who are dissatisfied with hard data and want to find a way to combine science and humanism. For many, giving up psychoanalysis is difficult because it seems to leave psychiatry dry and empty of meaning. This is the same problem that people have when they lose any form of faith. One can only hope that psychiatry will remain attractive as a discipline that addresses the great mysteries of the mind and of mental illness.

The Need for Belief and the Necessity of Doubt

Human beings have an almost universal need for belief. This psychological need is met by systems providing unified and coherent views of the world, and of the place of individuals in that world. Religion, socialism, and psychoanalysis share these characteristics. All are world-embracing systems of ideas that offer a complete account of the human condition. Theology, socialist thought, and psychoanalytic theory all claim to have discovered a hidden reality behind phenomenological appearances, the understanding of which can explain the inexplicable. Religion sees the experiential world either as an illusion or as a preparation for a future existence. Marxism tells us that whatever human motives seem to be on the surface, they are ultimately driven by class interests. Psychoanalysis also tells us that human motives are not what they seem, and that they derive from processes unavailable to conscious thought.

The most important supporters of psychoanalysis have been practising therapists. One can better tolerate the chaos of working with disturbed and difficult patients when one has a world view, particularly one that can explain much of what one sees. Other friends of psychoanalysis – intellectuals, humanists, and artists – live outside of the clinical world. In focusing on the creative and the irrational in life, analysis mirrors the trajectory of modernism. Basic elements of the analytic model have been used to explain the origins and impact of the arts, and have even created new hybrid disciplines such as psychohistory and psychobiography.[23] Yet few serious scientists have been supporters of psychoanalysis. An empirical training is a serious barrier to belief. Thus, the time when psychoanalysis dominated academic psychiatry can be seen as a non-scientific or pre-scientific era. Once medicine became linked to science, psychoanalysis was bound to fall into decline.

As the ideologies of the past century fade, and as both modernism and postmodernism play themselves out, science remains triumphant. Even non-scientists are fascinated with relativity theory and quantum mechanics. Evolutionary theory offers a model that can account for biological phenomena. One of the most important scientific advances of the twentieth century, the Watson-Crick model of DNA, has led to research mapping the genome, in which every intelligent person is interested, since it could lead to even more discoveries, from understanding the origins of life to treating incurable diseases. Medicine has made enormous strides, dramatically improving the treatment of infectious diseases and providing new hope for the mentally ill and their families. All these trends can only become stronger in the coming century.

The rise of psychoanalysis at the beginning of the twentieth century reflected the times; its decline reflects our own world. The decrease of religious belief and practice in developed countries has continued and even accelerated, gradually making a secular world view more normative. Gradually, people have become used to non-belief. As a result, there is less of a need for a replacement ideology than there was at the previous 'fin-de-siècle.' The crushing defeat of Marxism (and of other utopian political movements) has further reinforced scepticism about world-embracing ideologies.

Psychoanalysis suffered greatly from its arrogance. Having ridden so high, it was ripe for a fall. After claiming to explain phenomena in every sphere of knowledge, it may now be seen as explaining nothing. Scientific scepticism has becomes part of our intellectual culture.

Ideologies decline slowly over time. It has taken centuries for formal religious belief to decline; even so, ceremonial attendance is maintained when places of worship serve as sites for social networks. Many will continue to give lip service to faith, even as they reject specific theological tenets. Most traditional religious beliefs have been reinterpreted to meet the needs of the modern world.

A similar development has taken place in Marxism. The 'fundamentalist' belief in a classless society has almost disappeared. Instead, socialists prefer to speak of a fair redistribution of wealth and protection of the needy.[24] While this version of Marxist ideology is relatively bloodless, it retains a certain punch. Even today, its adherents can make headlines through demonstrations that disrupt international meetings.

Classical Freudian psychoanalysis is a relic of an earlier age, but revisionism has created newer versions of the old faith. To use a religious analogy, contemporary psychoanalysis resembles Norman Vincent Peale more than John Calvin. In this form, it could remain attractive for some time to come. At the same time, the vast array of therapies spawned by the psychoanalytic movement exert their own influence. The 'recovery movement' is a prominent example, since it unites religious and psychoanalytic themes into a potent and attractive mixture.[25]

By the end of the last century, Western civilization had witnessed the passing of many grand illusions. For most people religion has become more of an abstract principle than an ideology guiding the details of daily life. Many no longer require ultimate meaning, and are satisfied by the pragmatic empiricism of a life centred on work, family, and community. In the same way, political idealism has been transferred from a search for Utopia to practical and immediate goals. In personal therapy, the search for a 'complete analysis' has been replaced by the desire to function and to carry out a social role.

Can human beings ever live without illusions? The events of the last century have irreversibly reduced the strength and extent of many belief systems. The loss of religion's 'sacred canopy'[26] initially led to a search for other sources of ultimate truth, through either politics or personal therapy. Yet as substitute ideologies fail, living without them may become more normative.

In the coming century, fewer people will need to create a perfect world, and even fewer will want to achieve perfection in their personal lives. Medicine itself has to accept that there are limits to perfectability.[27] Psychiatrists today are more easily satisfied with a method such as psychopharmacology to control madness and depression, and with practical forms of psychotherapy whose efficacy is based on solid empirical evidence. The movement that Phillip Rieff described as introducing a 'therapeutic culture'[28] has been superseded.

One of Freud's greatest contributions to modern thought was the concept that human beings are more irrational than rational. Ironically, that very irrationality supported the creation of a psychoanalytic movement. Analysis survived because its supporters needed to believe. The question remains as to whether people will always require faith, or whether they can learn to live with uncertainty. At the centre of the scientific world view is *doubt*.

Notes

Introduction

1 Webster S. *Why Freud Was Wrong.* New York: Basic Books, 1995; Crews F. *The Memory Wars.* New York: New York Review of Books Press, 1995; Gellner E. *The Psychoanalytic Movement.* 2nd ed. London: Fontana, 1993; Macmillan M. *Freud Evaluated.* Cambridge, MA: MIT Press, 1997

2 Grunbaum A. *The Foundations of Psychoanalysis.* Berkeley: University of California Press, 1984

3 Hale N. *The Rise and Crisis of Psychoanalysis in the United States.* New York: Oxford University Press, 1995

4 Eisenberg L. Past, present, and future of psychiatry: personal reflections. *Canadian Journal of Psychiatry* 1997; 42:705–713

5 Ibid.

6 Hale, *Rise and Crisis of Psychoanalysis*

7 Ibid.

8 Beard R, Berlowitz L. *Greenwich Village: Culture and Counterculture.* Piscataway, NJ: Rutgers University Press, 1993

9 Auden WH. *In Memory of Sigmund Freud.* In: Mendelsohn E, ed. *Selected Poems of WH Auden.* New York: Random House, 1979

10 Hale, *Rise and Crisis of Psychoanalysis*

11 Rae-Grant Q, ed. *Images in Psychiatry: Canada.* Washington: American Psychiatric Press, 1996; Rae-Grant Q, ed. *Psychiatry in Canada: 50 Years (1951 to 2001).* Ottawa: Canadian Psychiatric Association, 2001; Naiman J. *A History of the Canadian Psychoanalytic Society.* Available at http://www.psychoanalysis.ca

12 Holt R, Luborsky L. *Personality Patterns of Psychiatrists.* New York: Basic Books, 1958; Henry WE, Sims JH, Spray SL. *The Fifth Profession.* San Francisco: Jossey-

Bass, 1971; Henry WE, Sims JH, Spray SL. *The Public and Private Lives of Psychotherapists*. San Francisco: Jossey-Bass, 1973; Menninger RW, Nemiah JC. *American Psychiatry after World War II, 1944–1994*. Washington: American Psychiatric Press, 2000

13 Menninger and Nemiah, *American Psychiatry*

14 Torrey EF. *Nowhere to Go: The Tragic Odyssey of the Homeless Mentally Ill*. New York: Harper and Row, 1988

15 English OS, Finch SM. *Introduction to Psychiatry*. 2nd ed. New York: Norton, 1960

16 For a summary of current knowledge, see Andreasen NC. *Brave New Brain: Conquering Mental Illness in the Era of the Genome*. New York: Oxford University Press, 2001

17 Dolnick E. *Madness on the Couch*. New York: Simon and Schuster, 1998

18 Hale, *Rise and Crisis of Psychoanalysis*

19 Freud S. The Question of Lay Analysis (1926). In: J Strachey, ed. *The Standard Edition of the Complete Psychological Works of Sigmund Freud*. London: Hogarth Press, 1956. 20: 179–258

20 Hale, *Rise and Crisis of Psychoanalysis*

21 Eysenck HJ. *Handbook of Abnormal Psychology*. London: Pitman, 1973

22 Dawes RM. *House of Cards: Psychology and Psychotherapy Built on Myth*. New York: Free Press, 1994

23 Eisenberg, Past, present, and future of psychiatry.

24 Dorwart RA, Chartock LR, et al. A national study of psychiatrists' professional activities. *American Journal of Psychiatry* 1992; 149:1499–1505

25 Dorwart et al, National study

26 Evidence-Based Medicine Working Group. Evidence-based medicine: a new approach to teaching the practice of medicine. *JAMA* 1992; 268:2420–2425; Sackett DL, Richardson WS, Rosenberg W, Haynes RB. *Evidence-based Medicine*. Edinburgh: Churchill Livingstone, 1997

27 Healy D. *The Creation of Psychopharmacology*. Cambridge, MA: Harvard University Press, 2002

28 Bliss M. *William Osler: A Life in Medicine*. Toronto: University of Toronto Press, 1999

29 Strachey J., ed. *Standard Edition of Works of Sigmund Freud*. London: Hogarth, 1955–64

30 Andreasen, *Brave New Brain*

31 Popper K. *Conjectures and Refutations*. New York: HarperTorch, 1968

32 Chessick RD. Psychoanalysis at the millennium. *American Journal of Psychotherapy* 2000; 54:277–290

33 Grunbaum, *Foundations of Psychoanalysis*.

34 Beck AT. *Cognitive Therapy and the Emotional Disorders.* New York: Basic Books, 1986

35 Sharfstein SS, Eist H, et al. The impact of third-party payment cutbacks on the private practice of psychiatry. *Hospital & Community Psychiatry* 1984; 35:478–481

36 Chipman A. Meeting managed care: an identity and value crisis for therapists. *American Journal of Psychotherapy* 1995; 49:558–67

37 Lambert M, ed. *Bergin and Garfield's Handbook of Psychotherapy and Behavior Change.* 5th ed. New York: Wiley, 2003

38 Malcolm J. *Psychoanalysis: The Impossible Profession.* New York: Vintage, 1982

39 Paris J. Canadian psychiatry across 5 decades: from clinical inference to evidence-based practice. *Canadian Journal of Psychiatry* 2000; 45:34–9

40 Goode E. Famed psychiatric clinic abandons prairie home. *New York Times,* June 2, 2003

41 Hollingshead A, Redlich F. *Social Class and Mental Illness.* New York: Wiley, 1958; Redlich F, Kellert SR. Trends in American mental health. *American Journal of Psychiatry* 1978; 135:22–28

42 Doidge N, Simon B, et al. Psychoanalytic patients in the U.S., Canada, and Australia: I. DSM-III-R disorders, indications, previous treatment, medications, and length of treatment. *Journal of the American Psychoanalytic Association* 2002; 50:575–614

43 Wallerstein R. *Forty-two Lives in Treatment.* New York: Guilford, 1986

44 Freud S. Analysis Terminable and Interminable (1937). In: Strachey, ed. *Standard Edition of Works of Freud.* 1968; 23:216–254

45 At www.apsa.org

46 Lambert, *Bergin and Garfield's Handbook*

47 Hale *Rise and Crisis of Psychoanalysis*

48 American Psychiatric Association. *Diagnostic and Statistical Manual of Mental Disorders,* 3rd ed. 1980.

Chapter 1: Psychoanalysis and Psychiatry

1 Sierles FS, Taylor MA. Decline of U.S. medical student career choice of psychiatry and what to do about it. *American Journal of Psychiatry* 1995; 152:1416–1426; Marcus SC, Suarez AP, Tanielian TL, Pincus, HA. Trends in psychiatric practice, 1988–1998: I. Demographic characteristics of practicing psychiatists. *Psychiatric Services* 2001; 52: 732–735

2 Hollingshead A, Redlich F. *Social Class and Mental Illness.* New York: Wiley, 1950

3 Henry WE, Sims JH, Spray SL. *The Fifth Profession*. San Francesco: Jossey-Bass, 1970

4 Harlow H, Woolsley CF. *Biological and Biochemical Bases of Behavior*. Madison: University of Wisconsin Press, 1958

5 Menninger RW, Nemiah JC. *American Psychiatry after World War II, 1944–1994*. Washington: American Psychiatric Press, 2000

6 Paris J, Kravitz H, Prince R. Report: Conference on key issues in post-graduate psychiatric education in Canada. *Canadian Journal of Psychiatry* 1986; 31:705–707

7 Lehmann HE. The future of psychiatry: progress – mutation – or self destruct? *Canadian Journal of Psychiatry* 1986; 31:362–367

8 Gabbard GO, Kay J. The fate of integrated treatment: whatever happened to the biopsychosocial psychiatrist? *American Journal of Psychiatry* 2001; 158:1956–1963

9 Hale R. *The Rise and Crisis of Psychoanalysis in the United States*. New York: Oxford University Press, 1995

10 Valenstein ES. *Great and Desperate Cures*. New York: Basic Books, 1986

11 Fink M. *Electroshock: Restoring the Mind*. New York: Oxford University Press, 1999

12 Collins A. *In the Sleep Room*. Toronto: Lester & Orpen Dennys, 1988

13 Shorter E. *A History of Psychiatry*. New York: John Wiley, 1998

14 Friedman L. *Menninger: The Family and the Clinic*. Kansas City: University of Kansas Press, 1998

15 Grinker RR, Spiegel JP. *War Neuroses*. Philadelphia: The Blakiston Company, 1945

16 Group for the Advancement of Psychiatry: see http://www.groupadpsych .org/about.html; Menninger and Nemiah. *American Psychiatry*

17 NIMH: see http://www.nih.gov/about/almanac/1998/organization/nimh/ history.html

18 Menninger and Nemiah, *American Psychiatry*

19 Hale, *Rise and Crisis of Psychoanalysis*

20 *American Journal of Psychiatry*, vol. 101, 1944

21 American Psychiatric Association, *Diagnostic and Statistical Manual of Mental Disorders*. Washington, 1952

22 Sackett DL, Richardson WS, Rosenberg W, Haynes RB. *Evidence-based Medicine*. Edinburgh: Churchill Livingstone, 1997

23 Gregg A. A critique of psychiatry. *American Journal of Psychiatry* 1944; 101:290

24 Dolnick E. *Madness on the Couch*. New York: Simon and Schuster, 1998

25 Bateson G, Jackson D, Haley J, Weakland J. Towards a theory of schizophrenia. *Behavioral Science* 1956; 1:251–255

26 Andreasen NC. *Brave New Brain: Conquering Mental Illness in the Era of the Genome.* New York: Oxford University Press, 2001

27 Dolnick, *Madness*

28 Freud S. A General Introduction to Psychoanalysis (1916). In: J Strachey, ed. *The Standard Edition of the Complete Psychological Works of Sigmund Freud,* vols. 15–16. London: Hogarth Press, 1963

29 Menninger K. *The Vital Balance.* New York: Peter Smith, 1963

30 Freud, General Introduction

31 Sullivan HS. *The Interpersonal Theory of Psychiatry.* New York: Norton, 1953

32 Fromm-Reichmann F. *Principles of Intensive Psychotherapy.* Chicago: University of Chicago Press, 1950

33 Green H. *I Never Promised You a Rose Garden.* New York: Holt, Rinehart and Winston, 1964

34 McGlashan T. *Schizophrenia: Treatment and Outcome.* Washington: American Psychiatric Press, 1989

35 Ibid.

36 Searles H. *Collected Papers on Schizophrenia and Related Subjects.* New York: International Universities Press, 1965

37 Semrad EV. Comprehensive therapy of schizophrenia. *Current Psychiatric Therapies* 1967; 7:77–81.

38 Arieti S. *Interpretation of Schizophrenia.* 2nd ed. New York: Basic Books, 1974

39 Will O. Schizophrenia and psychotherapy. In: J Marmor, ed. *Modern Psychoanalysis: New Directions and Perspectives.* New Brunswick, NJ: Transaction Publishers, 1968:551–573

40 Arietis S, ed. *Handbook of Psychiatry.* 2nd ed. New York: Basic Books, 1974

41 Bookhamer RS, Meyers R, Schrober C. A five year follow-up of schizophrenics treated by Rosen's direct analysis, compared with controls. *American Journal of Psychiatry* 1966; 123:602–604

42 Singer MT, Lalich J. *'Crazy' Therapies: What Are They? Do They Work?* San Francisco: Jossey-Bass, 1996

43 Planck M. *Scientific Autobiography, and Other Papers.* Chicago: University of Chicago Press, 1949

44 Dolnick, *Madness*

45 Levy J, Trossman B, Kravitz H, et al. Inpatients in love: conjoint therapy of two adolescents. *Canadian Psychiatric Association Journal* 1973; 18:435–438

46 May P. *The Treatment of Schizophrenia.* New York: Science House, 1968

47 Interview with John Gunderson, 24 April 2001

48 Gunderson JG, Frank AF. Effects of psychotherapy in schizophrenia. *Yale Journal of Biology and Medicine* 1985; 58:373–381

49 McGlashan TH. The prediction of outcome in chronic schizophrenia. *Archives of General Psychiatry* 1986; 43:167–176

50 Goldberg SC, Schooler NR, Hogarty GE, Roper M. Prediction of relapse in schizophrenic outpatients treated by drug and sociotherapy. *Archives of General Psychiatry* 1977; 34:171–184

51 Hogarty GE, Flesher S. Practice principles of cognitive enhancement therapy for schizophrenia. *Schizophrenia Bulletin* 1999; 25:693–708; Durham RC, Guthrie M, et al. Tayside-Fife clinical trial of cognitive-behavioural therapy for medication-resistant psychotic symptoms. Results to 3-month follow-up. *British Journal of Psychiatry* 2003; 182:303–311

52 Kernberg OF, Coyne L, et al. Final report of the Menninger Psychotherapy Research Project. *Bulletin of the Menninger Clinic* 1972; 36:1–275

53 Grinker RR. Editorial. *Archives of General Psychiatry* 1959; 1:1–2

54 Gedo E. Some difficulties of psychotherapeutic practice. *Archives of General Psychiatry* 1959; 1:3–6

55 Freedman A, Kaplan H. *Comprehensive Textbook of Psychiatry.* Baltimore: Williams and Wilkins, 1967

56 Sadock B, Sadock V. *Comprehensive Textbook of Psychiatry.* 9th ed. Baltimore: Williams and Wilkins, 1998

Chapter 2: Three Famous Universities

1 Rako S, Mazer H. *Semrad: The Heart of a Therapist.* Northvale, NJ: Jason Aronson, 1984

2 Leston Havens interview, 15 May 2001

3 Paul McHugh interview, 9 July 2001

4 Mack JE. *A Prince of Our Disorder: The Life of T.E. Lawrence.* Boston: Little, Brown, 1976

5 Mack JE. *Abduction: Human Encounters with Aliens.* New York: Ballantine Books, 1995

6 Sifneos PE. *Short-term Dynamic Psychotherapy: Evaluation and Technique.* 2nd ed. New York: Plenum, 1987

7 Lindemann E. Symptomatology and management of acute grief. *American Journal of Psychiatry* 1944; 100:141–148

8 Leon Eisenberg interview, 21 March 2001

9 Eisenberg L. Past, present, and future of psychiatry: personal reflections. *Canadian Journal of Psychiatry* 1997; 42:705–713; Eisenberg L. The past 50 years of child and adolescent psychiatry: a personal memoir. *Journal of the American Academy of Child & Adolescent Psychiatry* 2001; 40:743–748

10 Beam A. *Gracefully Insane: The Rise and Fall of America's Premier Mental Hospital.* New York: Public Affairs Books, 2001

11 Shervert Frazier interview, 16 May 2001

12 Meyers J. *Manic Power: Robert Lowell and His Circle.* Westminster, MD: Arbor House, 1987

13 Plath S. *The Bell Jar.* London: Faber and Faber, 1966

14 Kaysen S. *Girl Interrupted.* New York: Vintage, 1994; Nasar S. *A Beautiful Mind.* New York: Simon and Schuster 1998

15 Frazier interview

16 Kety SS, Rosenthal D, Wender PH. Mental illness in the biological and adoptive families of adopted individuals who have become schizophrenic. In: R Fieve, D Rosenthal, H Brill, eds. *Genetic Research in Psychiatry.* Baltimore: Johns Hopkins University Press, 1975: 147–165

17 Holzman PS. On the trail of the genetics and pathophysiology of schizophrenia. *Psychiatry* 1996; 59:117–127

18 Frazier interview

19 Available at http://www.carnegiefoundation.org/eLibrary; and see Fox DM. Abraham Flexner's unpublished report: foundations and medical education, 1909–1928. *Bulletin of the History of Medicine* 1980; 54:475–496

20 Osler W. *The Principles and Practice of Medicine.* New York: Appleton, 1898; Bliss M. *William Osler: A Life in Medicine.* Toronto: University of Toronto Press, 1999

21 McHugh PR. A structure for psychiatry at the century's turn: the view from Johns Hopkins. *Journal of the Royal Society of Medicine* 1992; 85:483–487

22 Kuhn T. *The Structure of Scientific Revolutions.* Chicago: University of Chicago Press, 1970

23 Shorter E. *A History of Psychiatry.* New York: John Wiley, 1998

24 Muncie WS. *Psychobiology and Psychiatry.* St Louis: Mosby, 1939

25 Hale R. *The Rise and Crisis of Psychoanalysis in the United States.* New York: Oxford University Press, 1995

26 Whitehorn JC, Betz B. Further studies of the doctor as a crucial variable in the outcome of treatment of schizophrenic patients. *American Journal of Psychiatry* 1960; 117:215–223

27 Eysenck H. The effects of psychotherapy: an evaluation. *Journal of Consulting Psychology* 1952; 16:319–324

28 Frank JD. Impressions of half a century at Hopkins. *Bulletin of the Maryland Psychiatric Society,* Feb 1995; 22(1)

29 Frank JD, Frank JB. *Persuasion and Healing.* 3rd ed. Baltimore: Johns Hopkins University Press, 1991

30 Lambert M, ed. *Bergin and Garfield's Handbook of Psychotherapy and Behavior Change.* 5th ed. New York: Wiley, 2003

31 Kanner L. Autistic disturbances of affective contact. *Nervous Child* 1943; 2:217–250

32 Kanner L. *A Word to Parents about Mental Hygiene*. Madison: University of Wisconsin Press, 1957

33 Bettelheim B. *The Empty Fortress*. New York: Free Press, 1967

34 Pollak R. *The Creation of Dr. B: A Biography of Bruno Bettelheim*. Carmichael, CA: Touchstone Books, 1997

35 Chakrabarti S, Fombonne E: Pervasive developmental disorders in preschool children. *JAMA* 2001; 285:3093–309

36 Hale, *Rise and Crisis of Psychoanalysis*

37 Hartmann H. *Ego Psychology and the Problem of Adaptation*. New York: International Universities Press, 1964

38 Mahler MS, Bergman A, Pine F. *The Psychological Birth of the Human Infant: Symbiosis and Individuation*. New York: Basic Books, 1975

39 Malcolm J. *In the Freud Archive*. New York: Diane Books, 1998

40 Federn P. *Ego Psychology and the Psychoses*. New York: Basic Books, 1952

41 Paris BJ. *Karen Horney: A Psychoanalyst's Search for Self-Understanding*. New Haven: Yale University Press, 1994

42 Roazen P. The exclusion of Erich Fromm from the IPA. *Contemporary Psychoanalysis* 2001; 37:5–42.

43 Rado S. *Adaptational Psychodynamics*. Northvale, NJ: Jason Aronson, 1969; repr. 1995

44 Kardiner A. *My Analysis with Freud*. New York: Norton, 1977

45 Sachar EJ. *Advances in Psychoneuroendocrinology*. Philadelphia: Saunders, 1980

46 Klein DF, Rabkin JG. *Anxiety: New Research and Changing Concepts*. New York: Raven Press, 1981

47 Donald Klein interview, 2 May 2001

48 Ibid.

49 Paul McHugh interview, 9 July 2001

Chapter 3: The Inner World of Psychoanalysis

1 Jones E. *The Life and Work of Sigmund Freud*. 3 vols. New York: Basic Books, 1953–7; Hale R. *The Rise and Crisis of Psychoanalysis in the United States*. New York: Oxford University Press, 1995

2 Kirsner D. *Unfree Associations: Inside Psychoanalytic Institutes*. London: Process Press, 2000

3 Kernberg OF. Thirty methods to destroy the creativity of psychoanalytic candidates. *International Journal of Psycho-Analysis* 1996; 77:1031–1040

4 Buckley P, Karasu TB, Charles E. Psychotherapists view their personal therapy. *Psychotherapy* 1981; 18:299–305

5 Janov A. *The Primal Scream.* New York: Putnam, 1970

6 Kirsner, *Unfree Associations*

7 Westen D. The scientific legacy of Sigmund Freud: towards a psychodynamically informed psychological science. *Psychological Bulletin* 1998; 124:360

8 Jones, *Life and Work of Freud*; Roazen P. *Freud and His Followers.* New York: Knopf, 1975

9 Paris BJ. *Karen Horney: A Psychoanalyst's Search for Self-Understanding.* New Haven: Yale University Press, 1994; Roazen P. The exclusion of Erich Fromm from the IPA. *Contemporary Psychoanalysis* 2001; 37:5–42

10 Alexander F, French T. *Psychoanalytic Therapy.* New York: Ronald Press, 1946

11 Grosskurth P. *Melanie Klein: Her World and Her Work.* New York: Knopf, 1986

12 Sullivan HS. *The Interpersonal Theory of Psychiatry.* New York: Norton, 1953

13 Paris J. The Oedipus complex: a critical re-examination. *Canadian Psychiatric Association Journal* 1976; 21:173–179

14 Strozier CB. *Heinz Kohut: The Making of a Psychoanalyst.* New York: Farrar, Straus and Giroux, 2001

15 Quinn S. Oedipus vs. Narcissus. *New York Times Magazine,* 9 November 1980: 120–126

16 Kohut H. *The Analysis of the Self.* New York: International Universities Press, 1970

17 Kohut H. *The Restoration of the Self.* New York: International Universities Press, 1977

18 Freud S. On Narcissism: An Introduction. In: J Strachey, ed. *The Standard Edition of the Complete Psychological Works of Sigmund Freud.* London: Hogarth, 1957. 14:67–102

19 American Psychiatric Association. *Diagnostic and Statistical Manual of Mental Disorders,* 3rd ed. 1980. Washington: American Psychiatric Press

20 Rogers C. *Counseling and Psychotherapy: Newer Concepts in Practice.* Boston: Houghton Mifflin,1942

21 Alexander, French, *Psychoanalytic Therapy*

22 Strozier, *Heinz Kohut*

23 Kohut H. The two analyses of Mr. Z. *International Journal of Psycho-Analysis* 1979; 60:3–27

24 Ragen BA. *Tom Wolfe: A Critical Companion.* Westport, CT: Greenwood, 2002

25 Lasch C. *The Culture of Narcissism.* New York: Warner, 1979

26 Paris J. *Social Factors in the Personality Disorders.* New York: Cambridge University Press, 1996

27 Kernberg OF. *Borderline Conditions and Pathological Narcissism.* New York: Jason Aronson, 1976

28 Jang KL et al. Heritability of personality traits: a twin study. *Acta Psychiatrica Scandinavica* 1996; 94:438–444

29 Frank JD, Frank JB. *Persuasion and Healing.* 3rd ed. Baltimore: Johns Hopkins University Press, 1991

30 Kernberg OF. The narcissistic personality disorder and the differential diagnosis of antisocial behavior. In: JR Meloy, ed. *The Mark of Cain: Psychoanalytic Insight and the Psychopath.* Hillsdale, NJ: Analytic Press, 2001: 315–337

31 Bowlby J. *Maternal Care and Mental Health.* WHO Monograph series # 2. Geneva: World Health Organization, 1951

32 Bowlby J. *Attachment and Loss.* 3 vols. London: Hogarth Press, 1969, 1973, 1980

33 Ainsworth MD et al. *Patterns of Attachment.* Hillsdale, NJ: Erlbaum, 1978

34 Cassidy J, Shaver PR, eds. *Handbook of Attachment: Theory, Research and Clinical Aspects.* New York: Guilford, 1999

35 Fink B. *A Clinical Introduction to Lacanian Psychoanalysis: Theory and Technique.* Cambridge, MA: Harvard University Press, 1998

36 Roudinesco E. *Jacques Lacan.* New York: Columbia University Press, 1993

37 Langs R. *Psychotherapy: A Basic Text.* New York: Jason Aronson, 1982

38 Armstrong K. *The Battle for God.* New York: Ballantine, 2001

39 Kardiner A. *My Analysis with Freud.* New York: Norton, 1977; Wortis J. *Fragments of an Analysis with Freud.* New York: Jason Aronson, 1984

40 Kovel J: *A Complete Guide to Therapy: From Psychoanalysis to Behavior Modification.* New York: Pantheon Books, 1976.

41 Jung CG. The Essential Jung. Ed. Anthony Storr. New York: MJF Books, 1996

42 Adler A. *The Neurotic Character: Fundamentals of a Comparative Individual Psychology and Psychotherapy.* San Francisco: Alfred Adler Institute of San Francisco, 2002

43 Perls F. *Ego, Hunger, and Aggression: The Beginning of Gestalt Therapy.* New York: Random House, 1969

44 Rogers CR: *Encounter Groups.* London: Allen Lane, 1971

45 See note 5 above.

46 Herman J. *Trauma and Recovery.* New York: Basic Books, 1992

47 Schacter DL. *Searching for Memory.* New York: Basic Books: 1996; McNally RL. *Remembering Trauma.* Cambridge, MA: Harvard University Press, 2003

48 Bass E, Davis L. *The Courage to Heal.* New York: Harper and Row, 1988

49 Merskey H. *The Analysis of Hysteria.* 2nd ed. London: Gaskell, 1995

50 Bloomberg D. Bennett Braun case settled; two-year loss of license, five years probation. *Skeptical Inquirer,* January 2000

51 Paris J. A critical review of recovered memories in psychotherapy: part I: trauma and memory. *Canadian Journal of Psychiatry* 1996; 41:201–205; A critical review of recovered memories in psychotherapy: part II: trauma and therapy. Ibid.: 206–210

52 Ofshe R, Watters E. *Making Monsters: False Memories, Psychotherapy, and Sexual Hysteria.* New York: Scribner, 1994; Showalter E. *Hystories.* New York: Columbia University Press, 1996

53 Crews F. *The Memory Wars.* New York: New York Review of Books Press, 1995

54 McNally, *Remembering Trauma*

55 Masson J. *The Assault on Truth: Freud's Suppression of the Seduction Theory.* New York: Farrar, Straus and Giroux, 1984

56 Malcolm J. *In the Freud Archive.* New York: Diane Books, 1998

57 See www.freedomforum.org/fac/90-91/masson91.htm

58 Masson J. *Against Therapy.* 2nd ed. Monroe, ME: Common Courage Press, 1994

59 Miller A. *Prisoners of Childhood: The Drama of the Gifted Child and the Search for the True Self.* New York: Farrar, Strauss, and Giroux, 1984

60 Merkin D. If only Hitler's father had been nicer. *New York Times,* 27 January 2002; review of Miller A. *The Truth Will Set You Free: Overcoming Emotional Blindness and Finding Your True Adult Self.* New York: Basic Books, 2001

61 Sobel D. A new and controverisal short-term psychotherapy. *New York Times Magazine,* 21 November 1982:51–58

62 Greenson R. *Technique and Practice of Psychoanalysis.* New York: International Universities Press, 1969

63 Kohut H. *How Does Analysis Cure?* Chicago: University of Chicago Press, 1984

64 Kandel ER. A new intellectual framework for psychiatry. *American Journal of Psychiatry* 1998; 155:457–469

65 Kandel ER. Biology and the future of psychoanalysis: a new intellectual framework for psychiatry revisited. *American Journal of Psychiatry* 1999; 156:505–524

66 Fonagy P, Target M. *Psychoanalytic Theories of Personality and Its Development.* London: Whurr Publications, 1999

67 Gabbard GO. *Psychodynamic Theory in Clinical Practice.* 3rd ed. Washington: American Psychiatric Press, 1999

68 Gabbard GO. Empirical evidence and psychotherapy: a growing scientific base. *American Journal of Psychiatry* 2001; 158:1–3

69 Brody AL, Saxena S, et al. Regional brain metabolic changes in patients with major depression treated with either paroxetine or interpersonal therapy: preliminary findings. *Archives of General Psychiatry* 2001; 58:631–640

Chapter 4: Counter-Revolution

1 Shorter E. *A History of Psychiatry.* New York: John Wiley, 1998
2 Kraepelin E. *Dementia Praecox and Paraphrenia.* Edinburgh: E. & S. Livingstone, 1919: 250
3 Kraepelin E. *Manic-Depressive Insanity and Paranoia.* Edinburgh: E. & S. Livingstone, 1921
4 Laing R.D. *The Divided Self.* Harmondsworth: Penguin, 1965
5 Schneider K. *Clinical Psychopathology.* Trans. M.W. Hamilton. New York: Grune & Stratton, 1959; Jaspers K. *General Psychopathology.* Vol. 1, trans. J. Hoenig and Marian W. Hamilton. Baltimore: Johns Hopkins University Press, 1999
6 Lewis AJ. *The Later Papers of Sir Aubrey Lewis.* Oxford: Oxford University Press, 1979
7 Mayer-Gross W, Slater E, Roth M. *Textbook of Psychiatry.* London: Ballier, Tindall and Cossell, 1960
8 Hudgens RW. The turning of American psychiatry. *Missouri Medicine* 1993; 90:283–291
9 RW Hudgens interview, 17 July 2002
10 Robert Cloninger interview, 13 December 2001
11 Robins LN. *Deviant Children Grown Up.* Baltimore: Williams and Wilkins, 1966
12 Robins LN, Regier DA, eds. *Psychiatric Disorders in America.* New York: Free Press, 1991
13 Guze S. *Why Psychiatry Is a Medical Specialty.* New York: Oxford University Press, 1992
14 Hudgens interview
15 Winokur G. Unipolar depression: is it divisible into autonomous subtypes? *Archives of General Psychiatry* 1979; 36:47–52
16 Andreasen, NC. *Brave New Brain: Conquering Mental Illness in the Era of the Genome.* New York: Oxford University Press, 2001
17 Tsuang MT, Tohen M, Zahner GEP. *Textbook in Psychiatric Epidemiology.* New York: Wiley-Liss, 1999
18 Cloninger interview
19 Roazen P. *Freud and His Followers.* New York: Knopf, 1975
20 Klerman G. Historical perspectives on contemporary schools of psychopathology. In: T. Millon, G. Klerman, eds. *Contemporary Psychopathology: Towards the DSM-IV.* New York: Guilford, 1986: 3–28
21 Muncie WS. *Psychobiology and Psychiatry.* St Louis: Mosby, 1939
22 See http://www.fda.gov/oc/history

23 Maser JD, Cloninger CR, eds. *Comorbidity of Anxiety and Depression*. Washington: American Psychiatric Press, 1990

24 Robins E, Guze SB. Establishment of diagnostic validity in psychiatric illness: its application to schizophrenia. *American Journal of Psychiatry* 1970; 126:107–111

25 Cooper JE, Kendell RE, Gurland BJ. *Psychiatric Diagnosis in New York and London*. London: Oxford University Press, 1972

26 Searles HF. *Collected Papers on Schizophrenia and Related Subjects*. New York: International Universities Press, 1965

27 Kraepelin E. *Manic-Depressive Insanity and Paranoia*. Edinburgh: E. & S. Livingstone, 1921

28 Andreasen, *Brave New Brain*

29 Kraepelin, *Manic-Depressive Insanity*

30 Muncie, *Psychobiology and Psychiatry*

31 American Psychiatric Association. *Diagnostic and Statistical Manual of Mental Disorders*. Washington: American Psychiatric Press, 1952

32 Menninger K. *The Vital Balance*. New York: Peter Smith, 1963

33 American Psychiatric Association. *Diagnostic and Statistical Manual of Mental Disorders*. 2nd ed. Washington: APA, 1968

34 World Health Organization. *International Classification of Diseases*. 10th ed. Geneva: WHO, 1992

35 Shorter, *History of Psychiatry*

36 See http://www.szasz.com

37 Szasz T. The Myth of Mental Illness: Foundations of a Theory of Personal Conduct. New York: Hoeber-Harper, 1961

38 Goffman E. *Asylums*. New York: Anchor, 1961

39 Scheff TJ. *Being Mentally Ill: A Sociological Theory*. 2nd ed. New York: Aldine, 1984

40 Rosenhan D. On being sane in insane places. *Science* 1973; 179:250–258

41 Laing RD. *The Politics of Experience*. London: Routledge & Kegan Paul, 1967

42 See http://www.decaelo.com/rdlaing/quotesby.htm

43 Burston D. *Wing of Madness: The Life and Work of R.D. Laing*. Cambridge, MA: Harvard University Press, 1996

44 Robins E, Guze SB: Establishment of diagnostic validity in psychiatric illness: its application to schizophrenia. *American Journal of Psychiatry* 1970; 126:107–111

45 Feighner JP, Robins E, et al. Diagnostic criteria for use in psychiatric research. *Archives of General Psychiatry* 1972; 26:57–63

46 Spitzer RL. An outsider-insider's views about revising the DSMs. *Journal of Abnormal Psychology* 1991; 100:294–296

47 American Psychiatric Association. *Diagnostic and Statistical Manual of Mental Disorders.* 3rd ed., Washington: American Psychiatric Press, 1980

48 *Diagnostic and Statistical Manual of Mental Disorders.* 3rd ed., rev., Washington: American Psychiatric Press, 1987

49 *Diagnostic and Statistical Manual of Mental Disorders.* 4th ed., Washington: American Psychiatric Press, 1994

50 *Diagnostic and Statistical Manual of Mental Disorders.* 4th ed., text revision. Washington: American Psychiatric Press, 2001

51 Shorter, *History of Psychiatry*

52 Goldberg D, Huxley P. *Common Mental Disorders: A Bio-Social model.* London: Tavistock/Routledge, 1992

53 Kisely SR, Goldberg DP. Physical and psychiatric comorbidity in general practice. *British Journal of Psychiatry* 1996; 169:236–242

54 Klerman GL, Weissman MM, eds. *New Applications of the Interpersonal Therapy of Depression.* Washington: American Psychiatric Press, 1993

55 Klerman GL, DiMascio, A. et al. Treatment of depression by drugs and psychotherapy. *American Journal of Psychiatry* 1974; 131:186–191

56 Elkin I, Shea T, Watkins JT, Imber SD. National Institute of Mental Health Treatment of Depression Collaborative Research Program: general effectiveness of treatments, *Archives of General Psychiatry* 1989; 46:971-982

57 Abrams R, Taylor MA. Importance of schizophrenic symptoms in the diagnosis of mania. *American Journal of Psychiatry* 1981; 138:658–661

58 Koehler KG, Steigerwald F. Consistency of Kurt Schneider-oriented diagnosis over 40 years. *Archives of General Psychiatry* 1977; 34:51–55

59 Ayer AJ. *Logical Positivism.* New York: Greenwood, 1978

Chapter 5: A Shrinking Perimeter

1 Shorter E. *A History of Psychiatry.* New York: John Wiley, 1998

2 Healy D. *The Psychopharmacologists.* New York: Chapman and Hall, 1997; and *The Psychopharmacologists III.* London: Arnold, 2000

3 Lehmann HE. Before they called it psychopharmacology. In: TL Sourkes, G Pinard, eds. *Building on a Proud Past.* Montreal: McGill-Queen's University Press 1995: 27–54

4 Valenstein ES. *Great and Desperate Cures.* New York: Basic Books, 1986

5 See http://www.healthyplace.com/Communities/Depression/ect/media/post.html

6 Lehmann H, Cahn CH, deVerteuil RL. The treatment of depressive conditions with imipramine. *Canadian Psychiatric Association Journal* 1955; 3:155–164

7 Shea MT, Elkin I, Imber SD. Course of depressive symptoms over follow-up. *Archives of General Psychiatry* 1992; 49:782–787

8 Gershon ES, Nurnberger JI. Bipolar illness. In: JM Oldham, MB Riba, eds. *Review of Psychiatry* 14. Washington: American Psychiatric Press, 1995: 405–424

9 Shorter, *History of Psychiatry*

10 Schou M, Baastrup PC. Lithium treatment of manic-depressive disorder: dosage and control. *JAMA* 1967; 201:696–698

11 May P. *The Treatment of Schizophrenia.* New York: Science House, 1968

12 Freud S. The Future Prospects of Psychoanalytic Therapy (1910). In: J Strachey, ed, *The Standard Edition of the Complete Psychological Works of Sigmund Freud,* London: Hogarth Press, 1957. 11:139–151

13 Elkin I, Shea T, Watkins JT, Imber SD. National Institute of Mental Health Treatment of Depression Collaborative Research Program: general effectiveness of treatments, *Archives of General Psychiatry* 1989; 46:971-982

14 Hollander E, Simeon D, Gorman JM. Anxiety disorders. In: RE Hales, SC Yudofsky, JA Talbott, eds. *The American Psychiatric Press Textbook of Psychiatry.* 2nd ed. Washington: American Psychiatric Press, 1994: 496–564

15 Freud. Notes upon a Case of Obsessional Neurosis (1909). In: *Standard Edition of Works of Freud.* 1955. 10:153–249

16 Casey DA. Obsessive-compulsive disorder: characteristic features, pharmacologic management. *Postgraduate Medicine* 1992; 91:171–174

17 Stein DJ. Obsessive-compulsive disorder. *Lancet* 2002; 360:397–405

18 Kossoff EH, Singer HS. Tourette syndrome: clinical characteristics and current management strategies. *Paediatric Drugs* 2001; 3:355–363

19 Klerman GL. The psychiatric patient's right to effective treatment: implications of Osheroff v. Chestnut Lodge. *American Journal of Psychiatry* 1990; 147:409–418; Stone AA. Law, science, and psychiatric malpractice: a response to Klerman's indictment of psychoanalytic psychiatry. Ibid.: 419–427

20 Stone AA. Where will psychoanalysis survive? *Harvard Magazine,* Jan.–Feb. 1997:34–39

21 Alan Stone interview, 6 May 2001

22 Leon Eisenberg interview, 28 March 2001

23 American Psychiatric Association. *Diagnostic and Statistical Manual of Mental Disorders.* 4th ed., text revision. Washington: American Psychiatric Press, 2001

24 T McGlashan, personal communication, 1988

25 Beck TA. *Cognitive Therapy and the Emotional Disorders.* New York: Basic Books: 1986

26 Aaron Beck interview, 1 August 2001

27 Kelly G. *The Psychology of Personal Constructs.* New York: Norton, 1955

28 Beck interview
29 Thorpe GL, Olson SL. *Behavior Therapy: Concepts, Procedures, and Applications.* London: Allyn and Bacon, 1997
30 Eysenck H. *The Effects of Psychotherapy.* New York: Science House, 1969
31 Eysenck H. The effects of psychotherapy: an evaluation. *Journal of Clinical and Consulting Psychology* 1952; 16:319–324
32 Wolpe J. *The Practice of Behavior Therapy.* 2nd ed. New York: Pergamon Press, 1973
33 Kennair LE. Behold the paradigm shift! *Human Nature Review* 2003; 3:196–209
34 Beck interview
35 Smith ML, Glass GV, Miller T. *The Benefits of Psychotherapy,* Baltimore: Johns Hopkins University Press, 1980: 10
36 Klerman GL, Weissman MM, eds. *New Applications of the Interpersonal Therapy of Depression.* Washington: American Psychiatric Press, 1993
37 Howard KI, Kopta AM, Krause MS, Orlinsky DE. The dose-effect relationship to psychotherapy. *American Psychologist* 1986; 41:159–164
38 Sifneos PE. Short-term Dynamic Psychotherapy: Evaluation and Technique. New York: Plenum, 1979; Mann J. *Time-limited Psychotherapy.* Cambridge, MA: Harvard University Press, 1973; Davanloo H. *Basic Principles and Techniques in Short-term Dynamic Psychotherapy.* Northvale, NJ: Jason Aronson, 1994; Malan DH. *The Frontier of Brief Psychotherapy.* New York: Plenum, 1976
39 Lambert M. *Bergin and Garfield's Handbook of Psychotherapy and Behavior Change.* New York: J. Wiley, 2003
40 At http://www.apsa.org
41 Zarin DA, Pincus HA, et al. Characterizing psychiatry with findings from the 1996 National of Psychiatric Practice. *American Journal of Psychiatry* 1998; 155:397–404; Olfson M, Marcus SC, Druss B, Pincus HA. National trends in the use of outpatient psychotherapy. *American Journal of Psychiatry* 2002; 159:1914–1920
42 Gabbard GO, Gunderson JG, Fonagy P. The place of psychoanalytic treatments within psychiatry. *Archives of General Psychiatry* 2002; 59:505–510
43 Bateman A, Fonagy P. Effectiveness of partial hospitalization in the treatment of borderline personality disorder: a randomized controlled trial. *American Journal of Psychiatry* 1999; 156:1563–1569; Bateman A, Fonagy P. Treatment of borderline personality disorder with psychoanalytically oriented partial hospitalization: an 18-month follow-up. *American Journal of Psychiatry* 2001; 158:36–42
44 Freud. Analysis Terminable and Interminable (1937). In: *Standard Edition of Works of Freud.* 1964; 23:216–254

45 Alexander F, French T. *Psychoanalytic Therapy.* New York: Ronald Press, 1946

46 Jong E. *Fear of Flying.* New York: Holt, Rinehart and Winston, 1973

47 Malcolm J. *Psychoanalysis: The Impossible Profession.* New York: Vintage, 1982

48 Sloane RB. *Psychotherapy versus Behavior Therapy.* Cambridge, MA.: Harvard University Press, 1975

49 Luborsky L, Singer B, Luborsky L: Comparative studies of psychotherapy: is it true that 'everyone has won and all shall have prizes'? *Archives of General Psychiatry* 1975; 41:165–180

50 Duncan BL. The legacy of Saul Rosenzweig: the profundity of the dodo bird. *Journal of Psychotherapy Integration* 2002; 12:32–57.

51 Wampold BE. Mondin GW, et al. A. meta-analysis of outcome studies comparing bona fide psychotherapies: empirically, 'all must have prizes.' *Psychological Bulletin* 1997; 122:203–215

52 Elkin et al., NIMH Treatment of Depression Program

53 Wampold E. *The Great Psychotherapy Debate: Models, Methods, and Findings.* Mahwah, NJ: Erlbaum Associates, 2001

54 Frank JD, Frank JB. *Persuasion and Healing.* 3rd ed., Baltimore: Johns Hopkins University Press, 1991

55 Strupp HH, Hadley SW. Specific vs. non-specific factors in psychotherapy. *Archives of General Psychiatry* 1979: 36:1125–1136

56 Strupp HH, Fox RE, Lesser K. *Patients View Their Psychotherapy.* Baltimore: Johns Hopkins University Press, 1969

57 Freud, Future Prospects of Psychoanalytic Therapy

58 At http://www.apsa.org

59 American Psychiatric Association. *Diagnostic and Statistical Manual of Mental Disorders.* 4th ed. Washington: American Psychiatric Press, 1994

60 Schneider K. *Clinical Psychopathology.* Trans. M.W. Hamilton. New York: Grune & Stratton, 1959

61 Sharaf M. *Fury on Earth.* New York: Da Capo Press, 1994

62 Reich W. *Character Analysis* (1933). New York: Farrar, Strauss, & Giroux, 1972

63 Reich W. *The Discovery of the Orgone.* New York: Orgone Institute Press, 1942

64 Paris J, ed. *Borderline Personality Disorder: Etiology and Treatment.* Washington: American Psychiatric Press, 1993; Paris J. *Borderline Personality Disorder: A Multidimensional Approach.* Washington: American Psychiatric Press, 1994; Paris J. *Personality Disorders Over Time.* Washington: American Psychiatric Press, 2003

65 Stern A. Psychoanalytic investigation of and therapy in the borderline group of neuroses. *Psychoanalytic Quarterly* 1938; 7:467–489

66 Grinker RR. *The Borderline Patient.* New York, Basic Books, 1968

67 Gunderson JG, Singer MT. Defining borderline patients: an overview. *American Journal of Psychiatry* 1975; 132:1–9

68 Maier W, Lichtermann D, Klingler T, Heun R. Prevalences of personality disorders (DSM-III-R) in the community. *Journal of Personality Disorders* 1992; 6:187–196; Torgersen S, Kringlen E, Cramer V. The prevalence of personality disorders in a community sample. *Archives of General Psychiatry* 2001; 58:590–596

69 Shea MT, Pilkonis PA, et al. Personality disorders and treatment outcome in the NIMH Treatment of Depression Collaborative Research Program. *American Journal of Psychiatry* 1990; 147:711–718

70 Gunderson JG. *Borderline Personality Disorder: A Clinical Guide.* Washington: American Psychiatric Press, 2001

71 Kernberg OF. *Borderline Conditions and Pathological Narcissism.* New York: Jason Aronson, 1976

72 Oldham JM, Gabbard GO, et al. Practice guideline for the treatment of borderline personality disorder. *American Journal of Psychiatry* 2001; 158 Supp: 1–52

73 Gunderson JG, Shea MT, et al. The Collaborative Longitudinal Personality Disorders Study: development, aims, design, and sample characteristics. *Journal of Personality Disorders* 2000; 14:300–315

74 Gunderson JG, Frank AF, et al. Early discontinuance of borderline patients from psychotherapy. *Journal of Nervous and Mental Diseases* 1989; 177:38–42

75 Linehan MM. *Cognitive-Behavioral Treatment of Borderline Personality Disorder.* New York: Guilford, 1993

76 Lehmann HE. The future of psychiatry: progress – mutation – or self destruct? *Canadian Journal of Psychiatry* 1986; 31:362–367

77 Luhrmann TM. *Of Two Minds: The Growing Disorder in American Psychiatry.* New York: Knopf, 2000

78 McHugh PR. The death of Freud and the rebirth of psychiatry. In: *The Weekly Standard Magazine,* Books & Arts, 17 July 2000

79 Martin L, Saperson K, Maddigan B. Residency training: challenges and opportunities in preparing trainees for the 21st century. *Canadian Journal of Psychiatry* 2003; 48:225–231

Chapter 6: Transition and Takeover

1 Brinton C. *The Anatomy of Revolution.* New York: Vintage, 1965

2 Fred Goodwin interview, 6 June 2002

3 Grinker RR. Psychiatry rushes madly in all directions. *Archives of General Psychiatry* 1964; 10:228–237

4 Draine J, Salzer MS, Culhane DP, Hadley TR. Role of social disadvantage in crime, joblessness, and homelessness among persons with serious mental illness. *Psychiatric Services* 2002; 53:565–573

5 Caplan G. *The Prevention of Mental Disorders in Early Childhood.* New York: Basic Books, 1961

6 Maier T. *Dr. Spock: An American Life.* New York: Harcourt Brace, 1999

7 Harmon RJ. The administration of programs for infants and toddlers. *Child & Adolescent Psychiatric Clinics of North America* 2002; 11:1–21

8 Steele MM, Wolfe VV. Child psychiatry practice patterns in Ontario. *Canadian Journal of Psychiatry* 1999; 44:788–792

9 Cohen L, Claiborn W, Specter GA, eds. *Crisis Intervention.* 2nd ed. New York: Human Sciences Press, 1983

10 Engel G. The clinical application of the biopsychosocial model. *American Journal of Psychiatry* 1980; 137:535–544

11 See http://www.nih.gov/about/almanac/1998/organization/nimh/history.html

12 Gibson RW, Cohen MB, Cohen R. On the dynamics of the manic-depressive personality. *American Journal of Psychiatry* 1959; 115:1101–1107

13 Wynne LC. Current concepts about schizophrenics and family relationships. *Journal of Nervous & Mental Disease* 1981; 169:82–89

14 Singer MT, Wynne LC. Principles for scoring communication defects and deviances in parents of schizophrenics: Rorschach and TAT scoring manuals. *Psychiatry* 1966; 29:260–288

15 Goodwin interview

16 Bunney WE. Drug therapy and psychobiological research advances in the psychoses in the past. *American Journal of Psychiatry* 1978; 135 Supp:8–17

17 Anonymous. Neurophysiologists honored (Ulf von Euler, Julius Axelrod, Bernard Katz). *Nature* 1970; 228:304

18 Robins LN, Regier DA, eds. *Psychiatric Disorders in America.* New York: Free Press, 1991; Kessler RC, McGonagle KA, et al. Lifetime and 12-month prevalence of DSM-III-R psychiatric disorders in the United States. *Archives of General Psychiatry* 1994; 51:8–19

19 Elkin I, Shea T, Watkins JT, Imber SD. National Institute of Mental Health Treatment of Depression Collaborative Research Program: general effectiveness of treatments. *Archives of General Psychiatry* 1989; 46:971-982

20 Goodwin interview

21 John Helzer interview, 8 May 2002

22 Helzer JE, Clayton PJ, et al. Reliability of psychiatric diagnosis. II. The test/retest reliability of diagnostic classification. *Archives of General Psychiatry* 1977; 34:136–141

23 Goodwin interview

24 Gunderson JG, Gabbard GO. Making the case for psychoanalytic therapies in the current psychiatric environment. *Journal of the American Psychoanalytic*

Association 1999; 47:679–704; Gabbard GO, Gunderson JG, Fonagy P. The place of psychoanalytic treatments within psychiatry. *Archives of General Psychiatry* 2002; 59:505–510

25 John Gunderson interview, 24 April 2001

26 Gunderson JG, Berkowitz C, Ruiz-Sancho A. Families of borderline patients: a psychoeducational approach. *Bulletin of the Menninger Clinic* 1997; 61:446–457

27 Gunderson, JG. *Borderline Personality Disorder: A Clinical Guide.* Washington: American Psychiatric Press, 2001

28 Joseph Coyle, personal communication, October 2002

29 McHugh PR. Witches, multiple personalities, and other psychiatric artifacts. *Nature Medicine* 1995; 1:110–114

30 Snyder S. *Drugs and the Brain.* 2nd ed. New York: W.H. Freeman, 1996

31 Lothstein LM. Sex reassignment surgery: historical, bioethical, and theoretical issues. *American Journal of Psychiatry* 1982; 139:417–426

32 Money J, Ehrhardt AA. *Man & Woman, Boy & Girl: The Differentiation and Dimorphism of Gender Identity from Conception to Maturity.* Northvale, NJ: Jason Aronson Inc., 1996

33 Colapinto J. *As Nature Made Him: The Boy Who Was Raised As a Girl.* New York: HarperCollins, 2000

34 DePaulo JR Jr, McMahon FJ. Recent developments in the genetics of bipolar disorder. *Cold Spring Harbor Symposia on Quantitative Biology* 1996; 61:783–789

35 Samuels J, Eaton WW, et al. Prevalence and correlates of personality disorders in a community sample. *British Journal of Psychiatry* 2002; 180:536–542

36 Allen Frances, personal communication, May 1994

37 John Oldham, personal communication, October 1999

36 Redlich F. *Hitler: Diagnosis of a Destructive Prophet.* New York: Oxford University Press, 1998

37 Hollingshead A, Redlich F. *Social Class and Mental Illness,* New York: Wiley 1950

38 Lidz T. *The Person, His and Her Development Throughout the Life Cycle.* Rev. ed. New York: Basic Books, 1976

39 Dolnick E. *Madness on the Couch.* New York: Simon and Schuster, 1998

40 Morton Reiser interview, 24 April 2001

41 Reiser M. *Memory in Mind and Brain.* New York: Basic Books, 1990

42 McGlashan TH. The schizophrenia spectrum concept: the Chestnut Lodge follow-up study. In: CA Tamminga, SC Schulz, eds. *Schizophrenia Research: Advances in Neuropsychiatry and Psychopharmacology.* New York: Raven Press, 1991; 1:193–200

43 Rosen JL, Woods SW, Miller TJ, McGlashan TH. Prospective observations of emerging psychosis. *Journal of Nervous & Mental Disease* 2002; 190: 133–141

44 Gershon ES. Bipolar illness and schizophrenia as oligogenic diseases: implications for the future. *Biological Psychiatry* 2000; 47:240–244

45 Eliot Gershon interview, 24 May 2002

46 Wallerstein R. *Forty-two Lives in Treatment.* New York: Guilford, 1986

47 Wallerstein R. Psychoanalysis: The Future of an Illusion? *International Psychoanalytic Association Newsletter* 1998, 7:1–5

48 Horowitz M. Stress-response syndromes. In: JP Wilson, B. Raphael, eds. *International Handbook of Traumatic Stress Syndromes.* New York: Plenum, 1993: 49–60

49 Marmar CR, Weiss DS, et al. Longitudinal course and predictors of continuing distress following critical incident exposure in emergency services personnel. *Journal of Nervous & Mental Disease* 1999; 187:15–22

50 Charles Marmar interview, 31 May 2002

51 Jambur Ananth interview, 16 July 2002

52 West LJ. A psychiatric overview of cult-related phenomena. *Journal of the American Academy of Psychoanalysis* 1993; 21:1–19

53 Ananth interview

54 Hendrick V, Altshuler L, Whybrow P. Psychoneuroendocrinology of mood disorders: the hypothalamic-pituitary-thyroid axis. *Psychiatric Clinics of North America* 1998; 21:277–292

55 Ananth interview

56 Naiman J. History of the Canadian Psychoanalytic Society, at http://www. psychoanalysis.ca

57 Cleghorn RA. The McGill experience of Robert A. Cleghorn. In: TL Sourkes, G Pinard, Eds. *Building on a Proud Past: 50 Years of Psychiatry at McGill.* Montreal: Department of Psychiatry, McGill University, 1994

58 Rakoff VM. The psychiatrist and the myth of the healer. *Canadian Journal of Psychiatry* 1992; 37(2):77–83

59 Leszcz. Integrated group psychotherapy for the treatment of depression in the elderly. *Group* 1997; 21:89–113

60 Segal ZV, Williams JMG, Teasdale JD. Mindfulness-based cognitive therapy for depression: a new approach to preventing relapse. *Psychotherapy Research* 2003; 13:123–125

61 P Garfinkel and A Kaplan, personal communication, 2002

62 Naiman, History of Canadian Psychoanalytic Society

63 Ibid.

64 Ackerman NW. Family psychotherapy today: some areas of controversy. *Jour-*

nal of Psychotherapy Practice & Research 1997; 6:151–164 (first published in 1966)

65 Miller IW, Kabacoff RI, Epstein NB, et al. The development of a clinical rating scale for the McMaster model of family functioning. *Family Process* 1994; 33:53–69

66 David Goldbloom, personal communication, 2001

Chapter 7: The Future of Psychoanalysis

1 Evidence-Based Medicine Working Group. Evidence-based medicine: a new approach to teaching the practice of medicine. *JAMA* 1992; 268:2420–2425

2 Mace C, Moorey S, Roberts B. *Evidence in the Psychological Therapies: A Critical Guide for Practitioners.* London: Brunner-Routledge, 2001

3 Nathan PE, Gorman JM: *A Guide to Treatments That Work.* 2nd ed. New York: Oxford University Press, 2002

4 Dixon RA, Munro JE, Silcocks PB: *The Evidence Based Medicine Workbook.* Boston: Butterworth-Heinemann, 1997.

5 Lambert M, ed. *Bergin and Garfield's Handbook of Psychotherapy and Behavior Change.* New York: Wiley, 2003

6 Schachter J, Luborsky L. Who's afraid of psychoanalytic research? Analysts' attitudes towards reading clinical versus empirical research papers. *International Journal of Psycho-Analysis* 1998; 79:965–969

7 Westen D, Morrison K. A multidimensional meta-analysis of treatments for depression, panic, and generalized anxiety disorder: an empirical examination of the status of empirically supported therapies. *Journal of Consulting & Clinical Psychology* 2001; 69:875–899

8 Festinger L. *A Theory of Cognitive Dissonance.* Stanford, CA: Stanford University Press, 1957

9 Frank JD, Frank JB: *Persuasion and Healing.* 3rd ed. Baltimore: Johns Hopkins University Press 1991

10 Sloane B. *Psychotherapy versus Behavior Therapy.* Cambridge, MA: Harvard University Press, 1975

11 Lambert, *Bergin and Garfield's Handbook*

12 Strupp HH, Fox RE, Lesser K. *Patients View Their Psychotherapy.* Baltimore: Johns Hopkins University Press, 1969

13 Wallerstein R. *Forty-two Lives in Treatment.* New York: Guilford, 1986

14 Eysenck H. *The Effects of Psychotherapy.* New York: Science House, 1969

15 Kernberg OF, Coyne L, et al. Final report of the Menninger Psychotherapy Research Project. *Bulletin of the Menninger Clinic* 1972; 36:1–275

16 Horwitz L. *Clinical Prediction in Psychotherapy.* New York: Aronson, 1974

17 Donald Klein interview, 2 May 2001

18 Dixon et al. *Evidence Based Medicine Workbook*

19 Strupp H, Hadley SW, Gomes-Schwartz B. *Psychotherapy for Better or Worse: The Problem of Negative Effects.* New York: Aronson, 1977

20 Lambert, *Bergin and Garfield's Handbook*

21 Shefler G. *Time-limited Psychotherapy in Practice.* New York: Brunner-Routledge, 2001

22 Gabbard GO, Gunderson JG, Fonagy P. The place of psychoanalytic treatments within psychiatry. *Archives of General Psychiatry* 2002; 59:505–510

23 Robert Michels interview, 6 August 2002

24 JC Perry, personal communication, 2002

25 Greenwald H. *The Call Girl.* New York: Ballantine, 1958

26 Paris J, Brown R, Nowlis D. Long-term follow-up of borderline patients in a general hospital. *Comprehensive Psychiatry* 1987; 28:530–535

27 Paris J, Zweig-Frank H. A twenty-seven year follow-up of borderline patients. *Comprehensive Psychiatry* 2001; 42: 482–487

28 Vaillant GE. *The Natural History of Alcoholism Revisited.* Cambridge, MA: Harvard University Press, 1995; Black DW, Baumgard CH, Bell SE. A 16–45 year follow-up of 71 men with antisocial personality disorder. *Comprehensive Psychiatry* 1995; 36:130–140

29 Kramer P. *Listening to Prozac.* New York: Viking, 1993

30 Freud S. Analysis Terminable and Interminable (1937). In: *The Standard Edition of the Complete Psychological Works of Sigmund Freud.* London: Hogarth Press, 1964; 23:216–254

31 Buckley P, Karasu TB, Charles E. Psychotherapists view their personal therapy. *Psychotherapy* 1981; 18:299–305

32 Gabbard G. *Psychodynamics in Clinical Practice: DSM-IV edition.* Washington: American Psychiatric Press, 1995

33 Malan DH. *Individual Psychotherapy and the Science of Psychodynamics.* Boston: Butterworth, 1979

34 Malan DH. *The Frontier of Brief Psychotherapy.* New York: Plenum, 1976

35 Luborsky L, Crits-Christoph P. *Understanding Transference: The Core Conflict Relationship Theme Method.* New York: Basic Books, 1990

36 Doidge N, Simon B, et al. Psychoanalytic patients in the U.S., Canada, and Australia: I. DSM-III-R disorders, indications, previous treatment, medications, and length of treatment. *Journal of the American Psychoanalytic Association* 2002; 50:575–614

37 Langs R. *Psychotherapy: A Basic Text.* New York: Jason Aronson, 1982

38 Erikson E. *Childhood and Society.* New York: Norton, 1950

39 Klein M. *Envy and Gratitude.* New York: International Universities Press, 1946

40 Bowlby J. *Attachment and Loss.* 3 vols. London: Hogarth Press, 1969, 1973, 1980

41 Westen D. The scientific legacy of Sigmund Freud: towards a psychodynamically informed psychological science. *Psychological Bulletin* 1998; 124:360–370

42 Grunbaum A. *The Foundations of Psychoanalysis.* Berkeley: University of California Press, 1984

43 Browne A, Finkelhor D. Impact of child sexual abuse: a review of the literature. *Psychological Bulletin* 1986; 99:66–77

44 Paris J. *Myths of Childhood.* Philadelphia: Brunner/Mazel, 2000

45 Harris JR: *The Nurture Assumption.* New York: Free Press, 1998

46 Rutter M, Rutter M. *Developing Minds: Challenge and Continuity Across the Life Span.* New York: Basic Books, 1993

47 Bowlby J. *Charles Darwin: A New Life.* New York: Norton, 1990

48 Malcolm J. *In the Freud Archive.* New York: Diane Books, 1998

49 Medawar P. Victims of psychiatry. *New York Review of Books,* 23 January 1975

50 Stone AA. Where will psychoanalysis survive? *Harvard Magazine,* Jan.–Feb. 1997: 34–39

51 Crews FC. *The Memory Wars.* New York: New York Review of Books Publishing, 1995

52 In: Crews, ibid.

53 *Time,* 26 November 1993

54 Crews FC, ed. *Unauthorized Freud: Doubters Confront a Legend.* New York: Viking, 1998

55 Vaughan S. *The Talking Cure: The Science behind Psychotherapy.* New York, G.P. Putnam's Sons, 1997

56 Westen, The scientific legacy of Freud

57 Brenner C. *An Elementary Textbook of Psychoanalysis.* Garden City, NY: Doubleday, 1957

58 Freud S. The Question of Lay Analysis (1926). In: *Standard Edition of Works of Freud.* 1956; 20: 179–258

59 Dawes RM. *House of Cards: Psychology and Psychotherapy Built on Myth.* New York: Free Press, 1996.

60 Gross PR, Levitt N, Lewis MW. *The Flight from Science and Reason,* New York: Academy of Sciences, 1997

61 Spence DP. The hermeneutic turn: soft science or loyal opposition? *Psychoanalytic Dialogues* 1993; 3:1–10

62 Maurice Dongier, personal communication

63 Leahy R. Cognitive therapy: current problems and future directions. In: RL Leahy, ET Dowd, eds. *Clinical Advances in Cognitive Psychotherapy: Theory and Application.* New York: Springer, 2002: 418–434

64 Robert Michels interview, 6 August 2002

65 Westen, The scientific legacy of Freud

66 Westen D, Gabbard GO. Developments in cognitive neuroscience: I. Conflict, compromise, and connectionism. *Journal of the American Psychoanalytic Association* 2002; 50:53–98

67 Andreasen NC. *Brave New Brain: Conquering Mental Illness in the Era of the Genome.* New York: Oxford University Press, 2001

68 Martin SD, Martin E, et al. Brain blood flow changes in depressed patients treated with interpersonal psychotherapy or venlafaxine hydrochloride: preliminary findings. *Archives of General Psychiatry* 2001; 58:641–648

69 Popper K. *Conjectures and Refutations.* New York: HarperTorch, 1968

70 Luhrmann TM. *Of Two Minds: The Growing Disorder in American Psychiatry.* New York, Knopf, 2000

71 Rogers C. *Counseling and Psychotherapy: Newer Concepts in Practice.* Boston: Houghton Mifflin, 1942

72 Greenberg LS. Evolutionary perspectives on emotion: making sense of what we feel. *Journal of Cognitive Psychotherapy* 2002; 16:331–347

73 Lambert, *Bergin and Garfield's Handbook*

74 Jaspers K. *General Psychopathology,* vol. 1. Trans. J. Hoenig and M.W. Hamilton. Baltimore: Johns Hopkins University Press, 1999

Chapter 8: The State of Contemporary Psychiatry

1 Guze S. *Why Psychiatry Is a Branch of Medicine.* New York: Oxford University Press, 1992

2 Mayberg HS, Liotti M, et al. Reciprocal limbic-cortical function and negative mood: converging PET findings in depression and normal sadness. *American Journal of Psychiatry* 1999; 156:675–682

3 Guze SB. Biological psychiatry: is there any other kind? *Psychological Medicine* 1989; 19:315–323

4 Engel G. The clinical application of the biopsychosocial model. *American Journal of Psychiatry* 1980; 137:535–544

5 Paris J. *Nature and Nurture in Psychiatry.* Washington: American Psychiatric Press, 1999

6 Monroe SM, Simons, AD. Diathesis-stress theories in the context of life stress research. *Psychological Bulletin* 1991; 110:406–425

7 Sierles FS, Taylor MA. Decline of U.S. medical student career choice of psychiatry and what to do about it. *American Journal of Psychiatry* 1995; 152:1416–426.

8 Robins LN, Regier DA, eds. *Psychiatric Disorders in America.* New York: Free Press, 1991

9 Shorter E. *A History of Psychiatry.* New York: John Wiley, 1998

10 Judd LL. The decade of the brain: prospects and challenges for NIMH. *Neuropsychopharmacology* 1990; 3:309–310

11 Paris, *Nature and Nurture*

12 Andreasen NC. *Brave New Brain: Conquering Mental Illness in the Era of the Genome.* New York: Oxford University Press, 2001

13 Meltzer HY. *Psychopharmacology: The Third Generation of Progress.* New York: Raven Press, 1987

14 Andreasen, *Brave New Brain*

15 Bradshaw R. Proteomics: boom or bust? *Molecular and Cellular Proteomics* (electronic journal), at http://www.mcponline.org

16 Kramer P. *Listening to Prozac.* New York: Viking, 1993.

17 Nedergaard M., Takano T, Hansen AJ. Beyond the role of glutamate as a neurotransmitter. *Nature Reviews Neuroscience* 2002; 3:748–755

18 LeDoux JE. *Synaptic Self: How Our Brains Become Who We Are.* New York: Viking, 2002

19 Bock G, Goode J. *The Limits of Reductionism in Biology.* New York: Wiley, 1998

20 Gray W, Fidler JW, Rizzo N, eds. *General Systems Theory and Psychiatry.* Boston: Little, Brown, 1969

21 Paris J. Evidence-based psychiatry: what it is and what it isn't. *Canadian Psychiatric Association Bulletin* 2002; 34:32–34

22 Stone AA. Law, science, and psychiatric malpractice: a response to Klerman's indictment of psychoanalytic psychiatry. *American Journal of Psychiatry* 1990; 147:419–427

23 Gunderson JG. *Borderline Personality Disorder: A Clinical Guide.* Washington: American Psychiatric Press, 2001

24 See Internet Mental Health, at http://www.mentalhealth.com

25 Fink M. *Electroshock: Restoring the Mind.* New York: Oxford University Press, 1999

26 Meltzer HY. *Psychopharmacology: The Third Generation of Progress.* New York: Raven Press, 1987

27 Healy D. *The Antidepressant Era.* Cambridge, MA: Harvard University Press, 1997

28 Meltzer, *Psychopharmacology*

29 Trivedi MH, Kleiber BA. Using treatment algorithms for the effective management of treatment-resistant depression. *Journal Clinical Psychiatry* 2001; 62 Suppl: 18:25–29

30 Lambert M, ed. *Bergin and Garfield's Handbook of Psychotherapy and Behavior Change.* 5th ed. New York: Wiley, 2003

31 Beck AT. *Cognitive Therapy and the Emotional Disorders.* New York: Basic Books, 1986

32 Eysenck HJ. *Handbook of Abnormal Psychology.* London: Pitman, 1973

33 Linehan MM. *Cognitive-Behavioral Treatment of Borderline Personality Disorder.* New York: Guilford, 1993

34 Crews F. *The Memory Wars.* New York: New York Review of Books Press, 1995

35 Kihlstrom JF. No need for repression. *Trends in Cognitive Sciences* 2002; 6:502

36 Crews, *Memory Wars*

37 Shapiro F, Maxfield L. Eye Movement Desensitization and Reprocessing (EMDR): information processing in the treatment of trauma. *Journal of Clinical Psychology* 2002; 58:933–946

38 Emmelkamp, PMG. Behavior therapy in adults. In: Lambert, M, ed: *Bergin and Garfield's Handbook*; 393–446

39 Shorter, *History of Psychiatry*

40 Linehan. *Cognitive-Behavioral Treatment*

41 Linehan, personal communication, 1997

42 Robert Michels interview, 6 August 2002

43 Wazana A. Physicians and the pharmaceutical industry: is a gift ever just a gift? *JAMA* 2000; 283:373–380

44 Beidel DC, Ferrell C, et al. The treatment of childhood social anxiety disorder. *Psychiatric Clinics of North America* 2001; 24:831–846

45 Zanarini MC, Frankenburg FR, et al. Treatment histories of borderline inpatients. *Comprehensive Psychiatry* 2001; 42:144–150

46 Paris J. *Personality Disorders Over Time.* Washington: American Psychiatric Press, 2003

47 Luhrmann TM. *Of Two Minds: The Growing Disorder in American Psychiatry.* New York: Knopf, 2000; Warme G. *The Cure of Folly: A Psychiatrist's Cautionary Tale.* Toronto: ECW Press, 2003

48 Schlesinger M, Wynia M, Cummins D. Some distinctive features of the impact of managed care on psychiatry. *Harvard Review of Psychiatry* 2000; 8:216–249

49 Lambert M, et al. Introduction and historical overview. In: *Bergin and Garfield's Handbook*

50 Torrey EF. *Nowhere to Go: The Tragic Odyssey of the Homeless Mentally Ill.* New York: Harper and Row, 1988

51 Lehmann HE. The future of psychiatry: progress – mutation – or self destruct? *Canadian Journal of Psychiatry* 1986; 31:362–367

52 Rosack J. September 11 underscores value of APA's mission. *Psychiatric News* 2001; 36:6–9

53 Bowman M. *Individual Differences in Post-Traumatic Response.* Mahwah, NJ: Lawrence Erlbaum, 1997

Afterword

1 Crossman RH, Engerman D, eds. *The God That Failed.* New York: Columbia University Press, 1955
2 Lerner D. *The Passing of Traditional Society.* New York: Free Press, 1958; Wellesz E, Sternfeld F, eds. *The Age of Enlightenment, 1745–1790.* New York: Oxford University Press, 1994
3 Bowlby J. *Charles Darwin: A New Life.* New York: Norton, 1990
4 At http://www.eecs.harvard.edu/~keith/poems/dover.html
5 Riley G. *Divorce: An American Tradition.* New York: Oxford University Press, 1991
6 Nietzsche F. *Thus Spake Zarathrustra.* Trans. Walter Kauffman. New York: Modern Library, 1995
7 Huyssen A. *After the Great Divide: Modernism, Mass Culture, Postmodernism.* Bloomington: University of Indiana Press, 1994
8 Koenig HG. Religion and medicine II: religion, mental health, and related behaviors. *International Journal of Psychiatry in Medicine* 2001; 31:97–109; Nooney J, Woodrum E. Religious coping and church-based social support as predictors of mental health outcomes: testing a conceptual model. *Journal for the Scientific Study of Religion* 2002; 41:359–368
9 Inglehart R, Baker WE. Modernization, cultural change, and the persistence of traditional values. *American Sociological Review* 2000; 65:19–51
10 Bender FL, ed: *Karl Marx, the Essential Writings.* 2nd ed. Boulder, CO: Westview Press, 1986
11 Gellner E. *The Psychoanalytic Movement.* 2nd ed. London: Fontana, 1993
12 Grotjahn M. Being sick and facing eighty. In: RA Nemiroff, CA Colarusso, eds. *The Race Against Time: Psychotherapy and Psychoanalysis in the Second Half of Life.* New York: Plenum, 1985: 293–302
13 Freud S. The Aetiology of Hysteria (1896). In: J Strachey, ed. *The Standard Edition of the Psychological Works of Sigmund Freud.* London: Hogarth Press, 1962; 3:191–224
14 Gellner, *The Psychoanalytic Movement*
15 Henry WE. *The Fifth Profession.* San Francisco: Jossey-Bass, 1971
16 Storr A, ed. *The Essential Jung.* Princeton: Princeton University Press, 1999
17 Peck MS. *The Road Less Traveled.* New York: Simon and Shuster, 1978
18 Stern K. *The Pillar of Fire.* Boston: Roman Catholic Books, repr. 2000
19 Adler A. *The Individual Psychology of Alfred Adler.* Ed. HL and RR Ansbacher.

New York: Basic Books, 1956; Paris BJ. *Karen Horney: A Psychoanalyst's Search for Self-Understanding.* New Haven: Yale University Press, 1994; Fromm E. *The Sane Society.* New York: Holt, Rinehart, Winston, 1955

20 Marcuse H. *Eros and Civilization: A Philosophical Inquiry into Freud.* Boston: Beacon Press, 1955; Brown NO. *Life Against Death: The Psychoanalytical Meaning of History.* Middletown, CT: Wesleyan University Press, 1959; Laing RD. *The Divided Self.* Harmondsworth: Penguin, 1965

21 Roazen P. The exclusion of Erich Fromm from the IPA. *Contemporary Psychoanalysis* 2001; 37:5–42

22 Sharaf M. *Fury on Earth.* New York: Da Capo Press, 1994

23 DeMause L. *Foundations of Psychohistory.* New York: Creative Roots, 1982; Volkan V, Itkovitz N, Dod AW. *Richard Nixon: A Psychobiography.* New York: Columbia University Press, 1997

24 Boaz D, Crane EH. *Market Liberalism: A Paradigm for the 21st Century.* Washington: Cato Institute, 1993

25 Mercandante LA. *Victims and Sinners: Spiritual Roots of Addictions and Recovery.* Louisville, KY: Westminster / John Knox Press, 1996

26 Berger PL. *The Sacred Canopy: Elements of a Sociological Theory of Religion.* New York: Bantam Doubleday Dell, 1990

27 Illich I. *Limits to Medicine: Medical Nemesis, the Expropriation of Health.* Toronto: McClelland and Stewart, 1976

28 Rieff P. *The Triumph of the Therapeutic: Uses of Faith after Freud.* Harmondsworth: Penguin Books, 1973

Interviews

Jambur Ananth, 16 July 2002
Aaron Beck, 1 August 2001
Robert Cloninger, 13 December 2001
Leon Eisenberg, 21 March 2001
Shervert Frazier, 16 May 2001
Elliott Gershon, 24 May 2002
Fred Goodwin, 6 June 2002
John Gunderson, 24 April 2001
Leston Havens, 15 May 2001
John Helzer, 8 May 2002
Richard Hudgens, 17 July 2002
Donald Klein, 2 May 2001
Donald Lipsitt, 6 August 2001
Charles Marmar, 31 May 2002
Paul McHugh 9 July 2001
Robert Michels, 6 August 2002
John Oldham, 9 April 2001
Morton Reiser, 24 April 2001
Alan Stone, 6 May 2001

Index